YOGA FOR
FOOTBALLERS

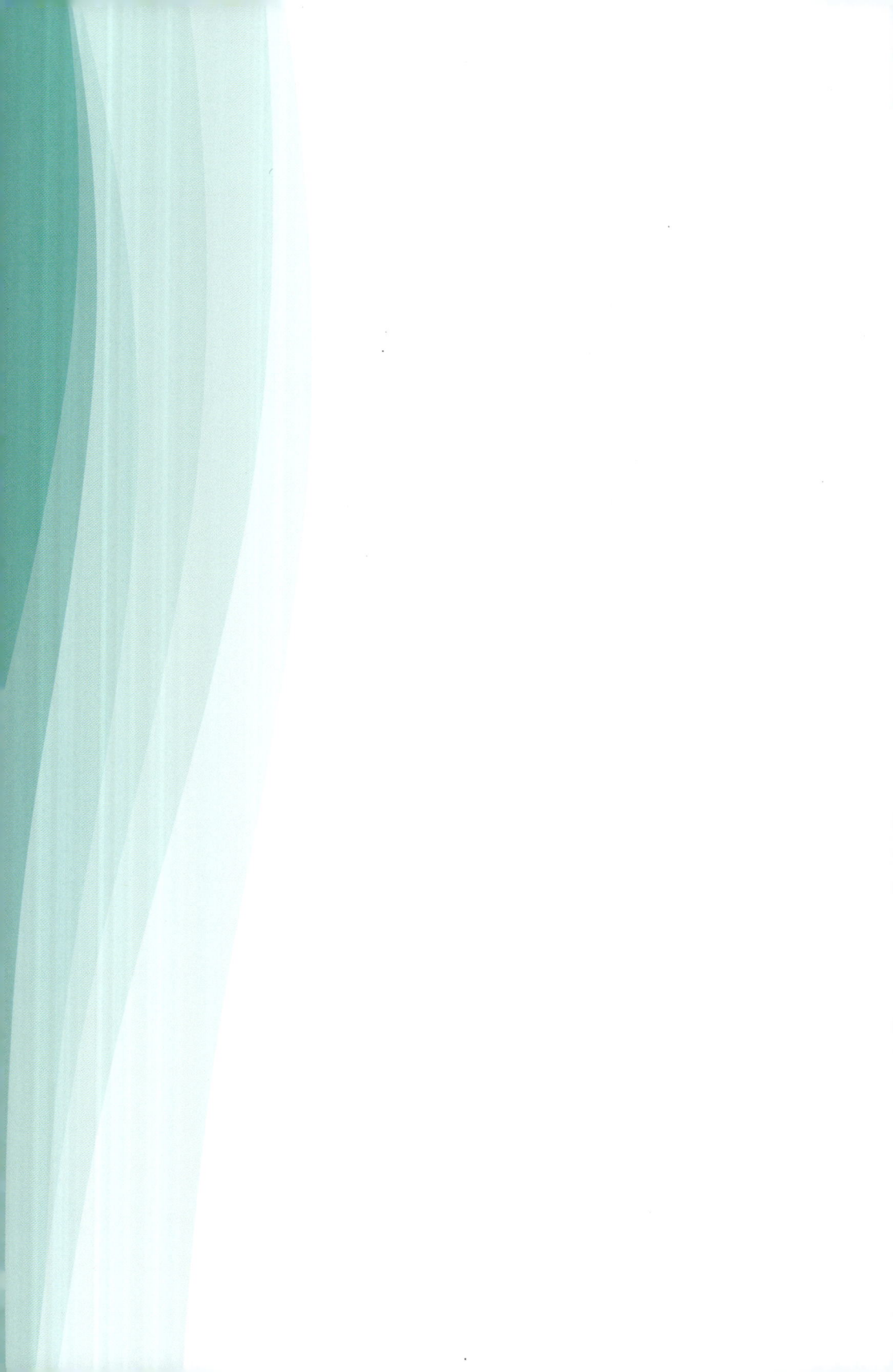

YOGA FOR FOOTBALLERS

MAXIMISE RECOVERY, PREVENT INJURIES AND PLAY BETTER FOR LONGER

Sharon Heidaripour

BLOOMSBURY SPORT
LONDON • OXFORD • NEW YORK • NEW DELHI • SYDNEY

BLOOMSBURY SPORT
Bloomsbury Publishing Plc
50 Bedford Square, London, WC1B 3DP, UK
Bloomsbury Publishing Ireland Limited
29 Earlsfort Terrace, Dublin 2, D02 AY28, Ireland

BLOOMSBURY, BLOOMSBURY SPORT and the Diana logo are
trademarks of Bloomsbury Publishing Plc

First published in Great Britain 2025

Copyright © 2025 Sharon Heidaripour

Sharon Heidaripour has asserted her right under the Copyright, Designs
and Patents Act, 1988, to be identified as Author of this work

For legal purposes the Acknowledgements on p. 158 constitute an extension
of this copyright page

All rights reserved. No part of this publication may be: i) reproduced or transmitted in
any form, electronic or mechanical, including photocopying, recording or by means of
any information storage or retrieval system without prior permission in writing from
the publishers; or ii) used or reproduced in any way for the training, development or
operation of artificial intelligence (AI) technologies, including generative AI technologies.
The rights holders expressly reserve this publication from the text and data mining
exception as per Article 4(3) of the Digital Single Market Directive (EU) 2019/790

Bloomsbury Publishing Plc does not have any control over, or responsibility for,
any third-party websites referred to or in this book. All internet addresses given in
this book were correct at the time of going to press. The author and publisher regret
any inconvenience caused if addresses have changed or sites have ceased to exist,
but can accept no responsibility for any such changes

Note: The information contained in this book is provided by way of general guidance
in relation to the specific subject matters addressed herein. The author and publisher
specifically disclaim, as far as the law allows, any responsibility from any liability, loss
or risk (personal or otherwise) which is incurred as a consequence, directly or indirectly,
of the use and applications of any of the contents of this book

A catalogue record for this book is available from the British Library

Library of Congress Cataloguing-in-Publication data has been applied for

ISBN (PB): 978-1-3994-1824-9
(epdf): 978-1-3994-1822-5
(epub): 978-1-3994-1825-6

2 4 6 8 10 9 7 5 3 1

All inside images © Henry Hunt (www.henryhunt.com) with the exception of the
following: pp. 11, 12, 13, 15, 16–17, 24–25, 31, 37, 41, 43, 45, 52, 56, 59, 62, 65, 68,
71, 82, 84–85, 101, 105, 109, 113, 117, 125, 133, 154 and 157 © Getty Images

Design by seagulls.net

Printed and bound in China by RR Donnelley Asia Printing Solutions Limited

To find out more about our authors and books visit www.bloomsbury.com
and sign up for our newsletters

For product safety related questions contact productsafety@bloomsbury.com

CONTENTS

Preface: Football, yoga and me   6
Introduction: Yoga and football   10

Part One: Essential daily routines
01 Morning routine   26
02 Pre-training/pre-match routine   40
03 Post-training/post-match routine   58
04 Evening routine   74

Part Two: Targeted routines
05 Hip routine   86
06 Hamstring routine   102
07 Lower back routine   118
08 Core routine   132
09 Relaxation routine   146

Sleep for peak performance   154

References   156
Acknowledgements   158
Index   159

PREFACE: FOOTBALL, YOGA AND ME

What sets my work apart is a profound understanding of the game. With over 35 years of experience, from playing to working as a professional physical therapist, I know how players move, feel and think, on and off the pitch. My holistic player-specific approach gives me the expertise to create and tailor sessions for the needs of individual players, reflecting on their current state, taking into account their training and match schedules, and overall wellbeing. This way of planning sessions makes sure players reach their absolute peak performance. My extensive background in football provides a unique perspective that other yoga teachers might not have. I understand the physical demands of the sport, the detailed and specific aspects of players' movements, and the psychological pressures they face both on and off the pitch, and on top of that I have myself experienced the highs and lows of a football career. I believe this provides me with unparalleled understanding and wisdom.

My love affair with football started when I was a toddler, playing out in the dusty streets of Rasht, in Iran, with the neighbourhood boys, dreaming of one day becoming a professional player. Then when I was eight, because of the war and the revolution in Iran, my family moved to Sweden. This was a pivotal moment in my life, and here I could finally join a girls' team and play for a club. From a young age I was a very talented player and was soon selected for one of the best teams in my region, then the county team, and eventually for a football high school, where I had the honour of winning the Swedish Youth Championship two years in a row. Football was my everything. I was determined to make it all the way to the top, and my dreams of a professional career were almost within reach. However, at 19, a serious knee injury shattered those ambitions.

The one thing I really loved had been taken away from me and I had to wait a long time before I could have surgery. I had lost my identity and didn't know who I was any longer. Depression had set in and I went into a downward spiral of bad company, alcohol, drugs and at times suicidal thoughts. That period, which lasted several years, was among the darkest of my life.

Looking back, if it wasn't for the love and support of my family, I don't think I would be alive today, because their unwavering love is what kept me going.

My physical health declined due to inactivity and I started to have other issues, like lower back problems, so I started to see a physiotherapist for both the knee rehab and my lower back pain. During these sessions, to help my back, I was introduced to certain yoga poses. The physio recommended that I went to yoga classes, so I did, and to my surprise I really enjoyed them. These classes not only made me feel stronger physically, but they also made me feel better mentally. After each session and on into the day after I felt lighter, happier and more alive.

Yoga helped me out of the darkness I was in. It helped me wake up and realise I loved football and really wanted to go back to it. Of course, I couldn't be a professional player now, but I could still make football my profession, so I found a BSc in Sports Therapy at London Metropolitan University, which looked perfect. Everything was related to sport and we learned about sports injuries, how to treat and rehab those injuries, and how to prevent them. I was very clear that my goal was to get back into professional football and with the Emirates Stadium being built next door to my university I had a vision that one day I would work at Arsenal Football Club.

BUILDING A CAREER IN FOOTBALL

I soon figured out I needed a good CV, so I reached out and applied for placements everywhere in football, so I could watch medical staff at work, learn from them and assist them. This helped me grow my contacts and my network, and every time I met someone new, I told them about my vision and that I was looking for more placement opportunities. Soon I was working with the London FA on youth match days, working alongside physios at non-league and semi-pro clubs all over the capital. I also qualified as a personal trainer and started my own business, working at gyms and also one to one with clients in their homes and in parks. The journey wasn't easy, but every challenge strengthened my determination.

In 2008, during my third year of university, I had a breakthrough, securing a placement at the Chelsea FC Academy. A few months into the placement I was offered a paid position at the club, which was surreal and a dream come true. My BSc was coming to an end, but I realised I wanted to study more and deepen my knowledge of football sports therapy, and I was so happy to find the perfect course, an MSc in Football Rehabilitation.

I loved the course, which was two years of part-time distance learning at Edge Hill University near Liverpool, and it was everything I had hoped for. It was football specific and covered all aspects of rehabilitation, performance, injury prevention, recovery and everything about what players needed on and off the pitch. I was living in North East London at the time, but had to travel to Liverpool every few weeks, and down to Cobham, to the Chelsea training ground, a few times a week, so I was constantly exhausted. However, since I pretty much lived around the corner from the Arsenal Academy training ground at Hale End, I decided to gamble and trust my instincts that everything was going to work out.

I handed in my notice at Chelsea and left the club in the middle of the 2010/11 season. My last shift with Chelsea was a Premier League tournament and all the teams up and down the country were taking part. I took the opportunity when we played Arsenal to tell their physios I had handed my notice in and to ask them to let me know if anything came up at the club. About a month later they got in touch. I had an interview and was offered a job. Working at Arsenal was always my ultimate goal, what I had been dreaming about all along, and reaching it was a significant milestone.

While at Arsenal I continued the private one-to-one work with clients. These were now mainly players I had worked with previously from the non-league clubs and Chelsea, and the work was more about performance, injury prevention and rehab. By now I had been practising yoga for several years and had really benefited from it, both physically and mentally. It seemed like a great idea to integrate it into my private work, so little by little I started to add certain poses, movements and breathwork techniques into my footballer clients' programmes.

Soon these same players, who were post-surgery, doing their rehab, were saying that they had never felt better or stronger, both in their bodies and minds. The yoga aspect of the training was allowing them to come back sooner from certain injuries, getting them out of that constant vicious cycle of playing a few games and then being out with an injury for a while. Integrating yoga into their programmes was also making them aware of what was going on with them physically and mentally, and allowing them to connect with themselves on a deeper level, physically, mentally and emotionally.

FOUNDING FOOTBALL YOGA

In 2015, after a few years of integrating yoga into my private work and being inspired by the astounding results, as well as having become a yoga teacher, I presented some examples of my success and my ideas about bringing this ancient practice to the players at the club to the academy's head of medicine and performance. Unfortunately, this was not something he was interested in, so in 2016 I took the bold step of resigning from Arsenal Football Club and founding Football Yoga. Although leaving Arsenal has so far been the hardest professional decision I have taken, I trusted my instincts because I knew in my heart of hearts that launching Football Yoga was the right path forward for me.

Football Yoga has since transformed the recovery and performance of players at every level, from the top flight to grassroots football. I have had the privilege of helping players who have gone through some of the most challenging times of their careers, dealing with serious injuries, and through Football Yoga I have been able to support them in their rehab and help them back to recovery and full strength. Traditional rehabilitation methods often overlook the mental and emotional aspects of recovery. Yoga addresses these gaps, offering a broad approach that enhances physical, mental and emotional

PREFACE: FOOTBALL, YOGA AND ME

resilience, and wellbeing, giving players the opportunity to be aware of the connection between their body and their mind and hence providing a more holistic and effective path to healing.

As a yoga teacher I have worked and supported players in the English Premier League, Championship, Leagues 1 and 2, and the leagues below, the Spanish La Liga, the French Ligues 1 and 2, and many other European leagues, as well as Major League Soccer in the USA and Canada, and players in Asian and Australian leagues. My unique approach, combining my deep understanding of football with the holistic benefits of yoga, has been featured in numerous prestigious publications, including *FourFourTwo*, *The Sun*, *The Mirror*, on Sky Sports, *The Athletic*, *GP* and *Aftonbladet*.

I currently live in Sweden and much of my work is done digitally, via Zoom. I have clients worldwide, of all levels and ages. I work directly with players or am connected to them via their agents or clubs, tailoring each session and programme to their specific needs. I also offer online Football Yoga injury prevention and recovery programmes and courses. Additionally, I deliver workshops, speak at events and also collaborate with football brands, app developers, magazines, coaches and others in the football industry to integrate Football Yoga into holistic health and wellness, further expanding the reach of my innovative approach.

MY PERSONAL JOURNEY

The journey from the streets of Iran to becoming a pioneer in football wellness has been anything but straightforward – I have needed resilience and adaptability – but every setback was the setup for a comeback, each challenge an opportunity for growth. There were triumphs and there were tears, but they all went into forming the professional I am today.

Through Football Yoga I strive to innovate, and to empower players to achieve their best holistic health and their optimal performance on and off the pitch. My story is one of transformation, a testament to the power of determination and the healing potential of yoga. It is a journey that highlights the importance of mental, emotional and physical wellbeing, and I hope that it inspires you and demonstrates that there is always a path to success, even during times of adversity.

As I look to the future, my vision remains clear: to change football's approach to wellness and holistic health by integrating yoga, breathwork and mindfulness. I want to ensure that players at every level and in every age group, especially the younger ones, have the tools they need to thrive, so this generation of players, and the ones to come, can have happier, healthier and longer careers.

My work is more than just a job; it is a passion, a calling and a commitment to excellence. Through innovation, dedication and a determined belief in the potential of holistic health, I continue to support those who love the game of football, proving that even in the darkest times new beginnings are possible.

Thank you for being here, for reading this book and for taking part in this journey.

Sharon Heidaripour
December 2024

INTRODUCTION: YOGA AND FOOTBALL

1. Why yoga and football are a good fit
2. What is yoga?
3. Six benefits of yoga for footballers
4. Yoga equipment
5. How to use this book

Yoga is an essential part of any footballer's toolkit. It balances your body and mind, supports healthy living and keeps you playing for longer.

INTRODUCTION: YOGA AND FOOTBALL

1. WHY YOGA AND FOOTBALL ARE A GOOD FIT

Cristiano Ronaldo, Lionel Messi, Kylian Mbappé, Michael Olise, Nikita Parris and Steph Houghton, along with other Lionesses squad players and the England's men's team, such as Harry Kane and Marcus Rashford. What do they have in common – apart from the obvious? The answer is that they, along with many other elite footballers, incorporate yoga into their training schedules. Some of them train with teachers at their clubs or while at tournaments, and some even have personal yoga coaches who train them one to one, in person or online.

Over the last decade, yoga has become more popular in a variety of sports, including football, but it's not just for those elite players. Footballers of all abilities and ages have become interested in yoga and what it can do for their game. You might be a youngster who loves playing for your school team and wants to be as good as you can be; perhaps you're a semi-professional playing in a lower league, who has started to feel a few aches and pains; or maybe you're a Sunday league player who just wants to keep turning out to play alongside your mates, despite your advancing years. On the other hand, you might not be a player yourself, but a match official, a coach, one of the medical staff who

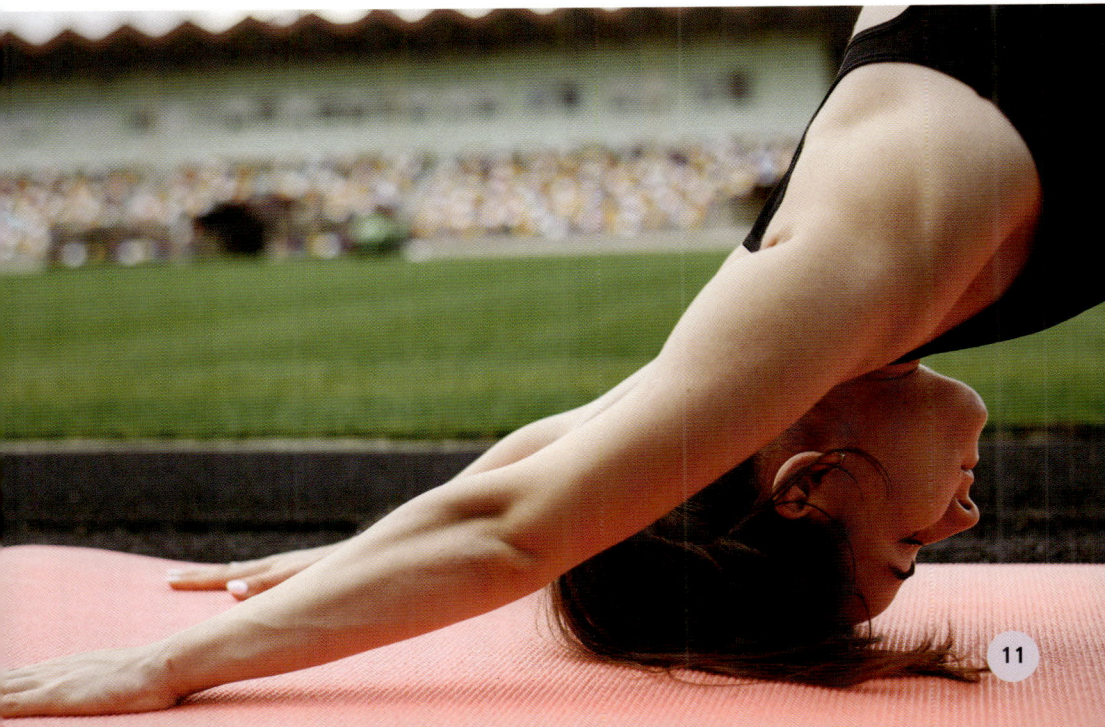

work in the sector or even the parent of a young player. Whatever your connection with the game, though, if you have at least a passing curiosity about the benefits of yoga for football, this book is for you.

THE ROOTS OF YOGA'S POPULARITY

These days we can connect with professional footballers on social media, following their lives on and off the pitch. Many share how they have overcome setbacks and injuries, often highlighting yoga's role in their recovery or crediting it for helping them maintain peak performance for extended periods. I also take great joy in seeing players celebrate their goals with yoga poses.

However, for a long time, yoga in football was seen as unconventional and even unsuitable. It wasn't until the legendary Manchester United and Wales player Ryan Giggs advocated for yoga and its benefits that it started to become more acceptable. Giggs began incorporating this ancient practice into his programme when he was in his late 20s, in the early 2000s. At the time he was dealing with recurring hamstring injuries and looking for alternative solutions to enhance his physical issues, and to extend his career. Giggs played in one of the highest ranked leagues in the world until he was 40. That is remarkable and he attributes much of his extended career, his high-level performance and the fact that he stayed relatively injury-free in the latter years of his career, to yoga.

Since those days, taking inspiration from Ryan Giggs, numerous clubs have integrated yoga into their training routines. Arsenal, Chelsea, Everton, Liverpool and Spurs, as well as European clubs such as Ajax, Bayern Munich, Juventus, PSG, and Real Madrid, and many others, have yoga teachers on their staff, for both their men's and women's teams. Some clubs even make this great resource available for their academy players.

Though initially its introduction was met with scepticism and it was seen as little more than a series of stretching routines, yoga in football has evolved and become the foundation of holistic player development. These days football clubs recognise the numerous benefits yoga offers their players, including physical fitness, injury prevention, recovery, and overall mental, emotional and physical wellbeing, and they are aware of how well it all complements their traditional strength and conditioning, rehab and prehab programmes. Yoga's impact on football goes beyond flexibility and physical recovery. It serves as a complete tool for enhancing a holistic state where players experience a balanced and harmonious integration of mental clarity, emotional resilience, physical health and career longevity.

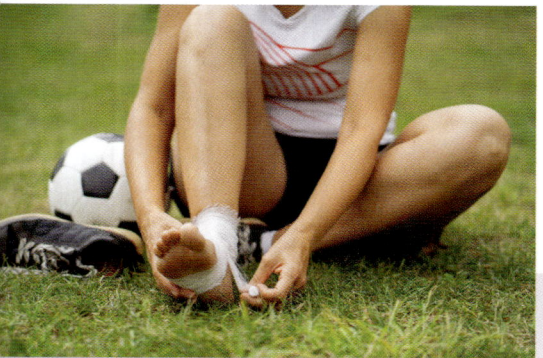

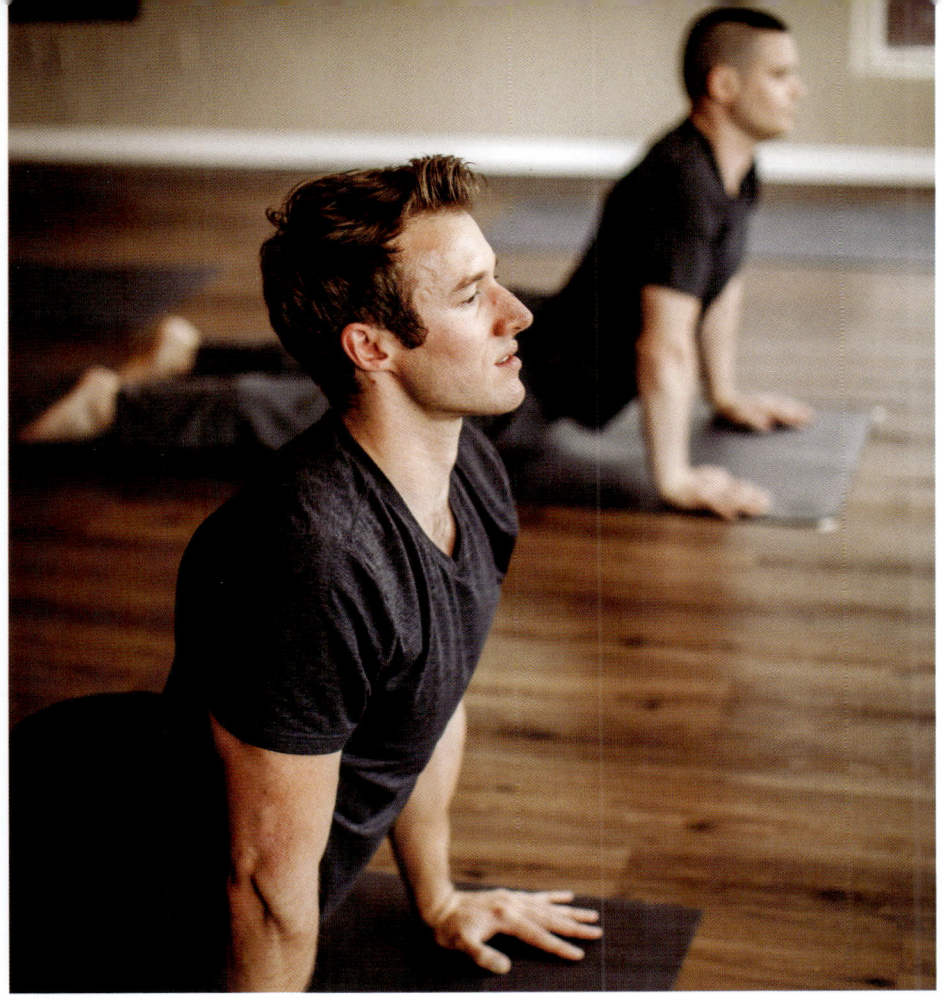

2 WHAT IS YOGA?

It's interesting that over the years of working in football, when I've asked people what yoga means to them, the answers vary. Many, for instance, describe it as 'stretching' or demonstrate meditation by touching their thumb and index finger together while making a humming sound. However, yoga encompasses much more than these aspects and serves as an umbrella term that means different things to different people, reflecting its diverse applications and profound depth.

Yoga is a complete science, a well-recognised discipline with principles and techniques, and a way of life that originated in India, and has been developed and practised for over 5000 years. It made its way to the West in the late 19th century and has since become a widespread holistic practice that encourages personal growth, ethical living and a balanced approach to health, wellbeing and life. It is a multifaceted yet integrated system that addresses our body, mind, emotions and inner self, allowing us to develop a deeper connection with ourselves and the world around us, and encouraging a sense of oneness and peace.

Yoga goes beyond mere physical postures, it also integrates meditation, ethical principles, practices aimed at self-awareness and breathing techniques. Though yoga may include spiritual elements like mindfulness and meditation, it is not a religion, and its practice is not limited to any specific religious context, making it inclusive and open to everyone. Yoga can be practised by individuals of any faith or those without religious beliefs, and is practised not only by Hindus but also Muslims, Buddhists, Jews and Christians all over the world – the word 'yoga' has its origins in the Sanskrit language meaning 'to join' or 'to unite'.

PHYSICAL POSES

Yoga poses – called asanas – offer a wide range of benefits that extend beyond physical fitness, as they enhance mental wellbeing and promote a stronger connection between the body and mind. Whether you're a beginner or have been practising for a long time, yoga adapts to meet your individual needs. Integrating yoga and movement into your daily life is great for waking up the body, being in the present moment and finding focus when your brain is over-stimulated – crucial at high-pressure points throughout the season.

BREATHWORK

We seldom pay attention to it in our everyday life, but the rhythm and depth of our breath mirrors our state of mind. When we are stressed, our breath is shallow and fast, and when we are calm our breath is deep and slow. By noticing and observing our breath we can deepen our awareness of how we are feeling in the now, and although breath is always involuntary we can still consciously control it and slow it down.

When we breathe deeply and consciously, the parasympathetic nervous system, our rest and digest system, is stimulated. This helps our body to relax, lowers our stress levels and increases the flow of oxygen, which in turn increases our energy levels and improves our focus. There are different techniques for controlling the breath – called pranayamas – some of which are shared in this book. They will improve your calmness, mental clarity and endurance, enhancing your performance and enabling you to stay on top of your game.

NOTE
The poses in this book have been modified, based on my experience, to better suit the needs of footballers. I have also adapted or invented some of the names of exercises, so even though you're a regular yogi you may not have encountered them before or you might know them by other names.

INTRODUCTION: YOGA AND FOOTBALL

YOGA VERSUS STRETCHING

I am often asked about the differences between yoga and stretching, and over the years I have come across football players who say, 'I don't do yoga because I've heard stretching reduces muscle power.' Yes, if you stretch a muscle too much it isn't good for the muscle's health, especially before training or a match. However, yoga is not about damaging your body, it's about empowering it. Let me explain.

Stretching involves elongating specific muscles to increase flexibility and range of motion. This temporarily lengthens muscle fibres and improves elasticity. However, stretching too much, particularly before a game or training, can decrease muscle tone and power output. It may disrupt the muscle's optimal length-tension relationship, which is fundamental for peak performance.

Lengthening, by contrast, focuses on enhancing overall muscle and fascial function. This approach includes exercises, like yoga, designed to improve balance and posture by engaging the body's myofascial system, which consists of muscles, fascia, tendons and ligaments. The aim is to enhance the functional length and alignment of the entire chain of muscles and fascia. By targeting this complete chain, lengthening promotes balanced muscle activation without the loss of power and strength.

In yoga, the emphasis is primarily on lengthening the body, unlike traditional stretching that targets specific muscles. This method supports improved flexibility and strength without compromising power. Even though yoga combines static and dynamic stretches, the postures work with the whole body, rather than isolated muscle groups.

For footballers, understanding these differences is crucial. Dynamic stretching and movements should be included before training and games to prepare muscles without reducing power. Conversely, static stretching is more beneficial after matches or training, as it encourages muscle relaxation and recovery.

The key is to balance flexibility with strength, ensuring that muscles remain flexible yet powerful throughout their entire range of motion. The postures, movements and exercises in this book are based on these principles.

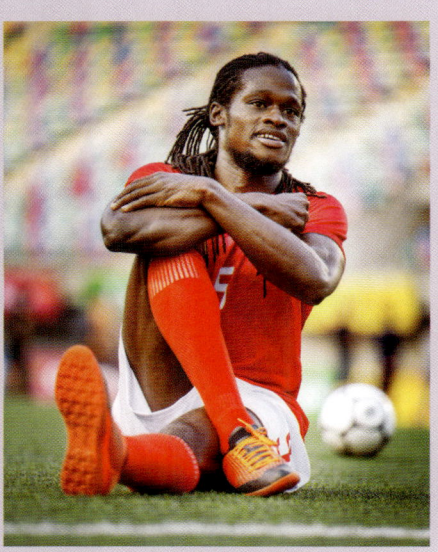

3 SIX BENEFITS OF YOGA FOR FOOTBALLERS

1 IMPROVED MUSCLE FLEXIBILITY

Yoga includes a range of static stretches and dynamic movements that lengthen muscles and enhance elasticity, which is crucial for improving overall flexibility. This flexibility is essential for footballers, who need to execute quick and agile movements on the pitch. Flexible muscles contract more effectively, resulting in increased power for actions such as sprinting, jumping and shooting, while also allowing for more fluid and dynamic movements.

Research published in the *International Journal of Yoga* supports these benefits, highlighting the positive impact of yoga on muscle flexibility, particularly in the hip region. A study of 26 athletes following a structured yoga programme over a 10-week period documented significant improvements in hip flexibility and overall muscle performance. Poses like downward-facing dog (see page 48), low lunge cactus arms (see page 123) and pigeon (see page 79) are particularly effective for enhancing flexibility in the back, front line of the body and hips, further emphasising yoga's value in athletic training.

2 ENHANCED JOINT MOBILITY AND STABILITY

Beyond flexibility, yoga also increases the range of motion in the joints, and strengthens and lengthens the muscles around them, helping players maintain joint stability and achieve a wider range of movement. The same study, published in the *International Journal of Yoga*, further suggests that yoga significantly improves the range of motion and functional performance in athletes. The research highlights that yoga enhances joint mobility, angles, flexibility and balance in key areas such as the hips, shoulders and ankles, contributing to better agility and stability on the pitch. Stable joints are better equipped to handle the stresses of quick changes and impacts, while an increased range of motion is crucial for jumping, pivoting and kicking. Poses like cat and cow (see page 28)

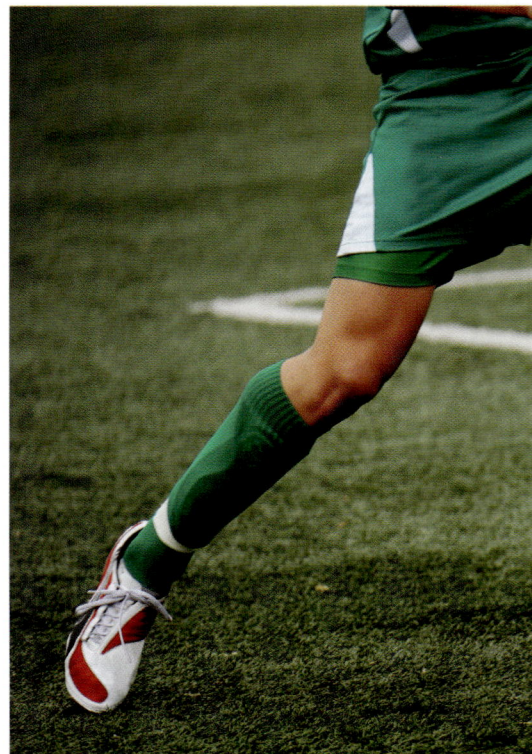

and thread the needle (see page 121) enhance spinal mobility, while poses such as warrior 3 (see page 53) and football star (see page 54) support hip, knee and ankle joint stability, helping to prevent injuries in these critical areas.

3 EFFICIENT RECOVERY

Yoga's important role in mental and physical recovery cannot be exaggerated. According to a 2023 study published in the *International Journal of Yoga*, yoga significantly enhances recovery after high-intensity exercise. It helps players restore strength, balance and flexibility while improving circulation, and also boosts oxygen supply to tissues, enabling players to recover better and regain optimal performance.

Additionally, yoga's relaxation and mindfulness components support mental recovery by reducing stress and improving sleep quality, both of which are crucial for overall physical recovery. The postures in the post-training/post-match routine are excellent for facilitating the removal of lactic acid and other toxins. When combined with the evening routine and relaxation routine, gentle restorative poses such as legs up the wall (see page 81) and child's pose (see page 80), along with practices like bananasana (see page 153) and various breathing exercises (see page 148), are effective for calming both the body and mind, contributing to a more comprehensive recovery process.

4 ENHANCED PERFORMANCE

Yoga provides numerous benefits that directly enhance football performance by improving flexibility and mobility, leading to better agility and coordination. This results in more fluid and precise responses to the fast-paced and unpredictable nature of football. Strengthening core and lower body muscles through yoga creates a solid basis for stability, enabling more powerful and explosive movements on the pitch. Regular practice of yoga enhances muscle function and energy transfer, which contributes to increased endurance, strength and power while lowering the risk of injury.

In a study published in the *International Journal of Human Movement and Sports Sciences*, a six-week yoga programme incorporating some of the exercises in this book, practised four times a week, demonstrated significant improvements in achieving peak performance levels for footballers. The programme positively supported motor development, including strength, balance and flexibility. The study also suggested that a yoga routine could serve as an effective alternative for coaches to include in their training programmes. This research underscores the value of incorporating yoga into athletic training programmes to enhance balance, flexibility, strength and overall performance. Poses like sun salutation (see page 34) and the one-legged dog flow (see page 142) are particularly effective in enhancing movement fluidity and creating a strong foundation for explosive actions on the pitch.

5 INJURY PREVENTION

Yoga is increasingly recognised as a crucial element in footballers' training schedules due to its effectiveness in preventing injuries. One of its primary benefits is promoting muscle balance by evenly strengthening and lengthening all muscle groups, which helps prevent imbalances that can lead to injury. Balanced muscle development ensures that load is distributed evenly, reducing the risk of muscular strains. Poses like bridge (see page 124), tree (see page 98) and warrior 2 (see page 145) are particularly effective in maintaining muscle symmetry.

Additionally, yoga strengthens and stretches soft tissues, including ligaments, tendons and facia, increasing their resilience to the demands of the game. This enhances overall joint stability, helping to prevent ligament tears and sprains, tendon tears and overuse injuries. A study in 2020 published in the *International Journal of Yoga* examined the impact of yoga on mitigating the causes that contribute to sports-related injuries.

The research found that a 10-week yoga intervention for football players helped reduce key elements like perceived injury risk and fatigue, which are known to increase injury susceptibility. These findings suggest that yoga can play a significant role in preventing injuries by addressing stress-related factors and enhancing overall player wellbeing.

6 MENTAL FOCUS AND RELAXATION

By incorporating mindfulness and breathing techniques from yoga, footballers can manage stress, enhance concentration and maintain mental clarity during high-pressure situations in a game. In an article published in *Brain Plasticity*, a systematic review of the literature revealed evidence that yoga can positively impact brain health. Although the study was not specifically targeted at athletes, it highlighted that yoga could improve focus, stress regulation and cognitive performance, which are benefits that are highly relevant to athletic performance.

Yoga also promotes relaxation and helps reduce anxiety, contributing to better sleep quality. Sufficient rest is crucial for players to recover effectively, and maintain peak physical and mental performance throughout the season. Breathing exercises such as alternate nostril breathing (see page 149) and the 4-7-8 technique (see page 83), along with any of the restorative poses in this book, are particularly effective for enhancing relaxation in both the body and mind, and for improving mental focus.

INTRODUCTION: YOGA AND FOOTBALL

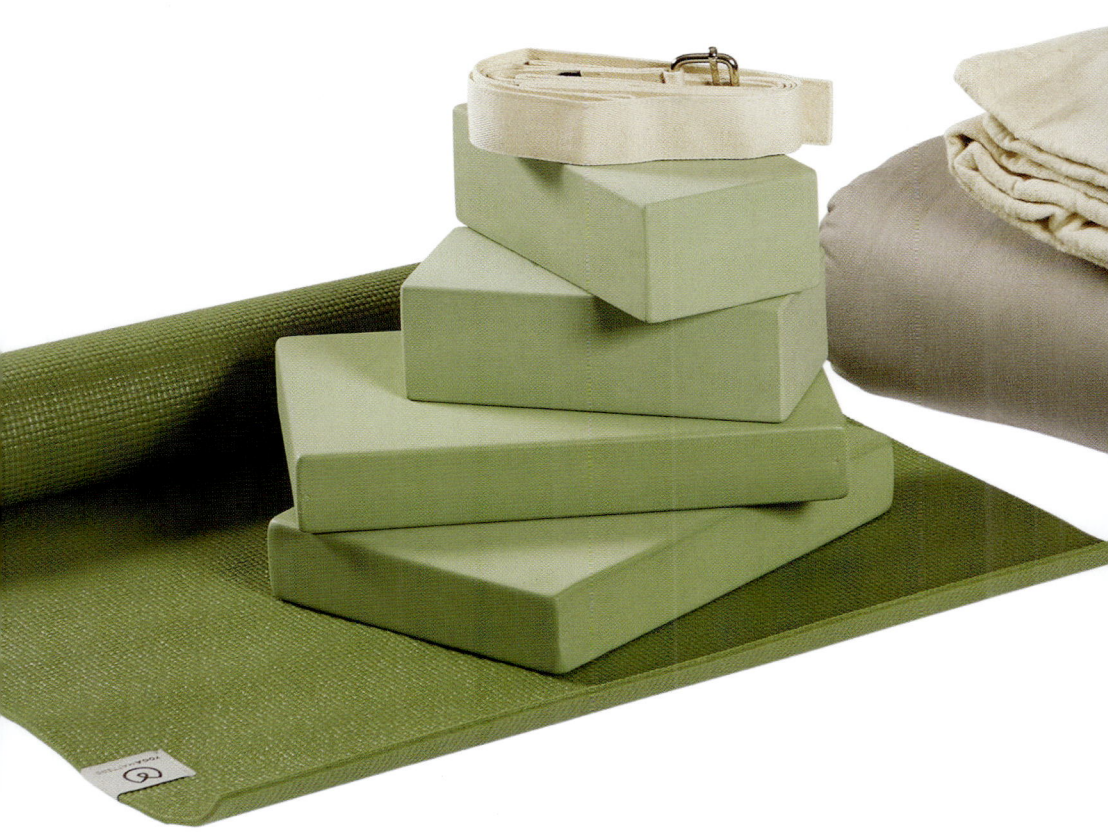

4 YOGA EQUIPMENT

Specific yoga equipment isn't essential, but it is helpful, especially when you're a beginner or have physical limitations. It will help you maintain good alignment and posture, and help you to practise safely, providing you with support and comfort. Having appropriate clothing is also important when practising yoga. Any type of activewear that you feel comfortable in – that is breathable, flexible and non-restrictive – is a great option. It is advisable to practise without socks to avoid slipping, however if you wish to wear some, you can find some with grips and rubber soles. You can always wear your trainers as well, it is a personal choice, but practising barefoot fosters sensory awareness, brings you greater strength and improves balance. I always encourage clients to practise barefoot.

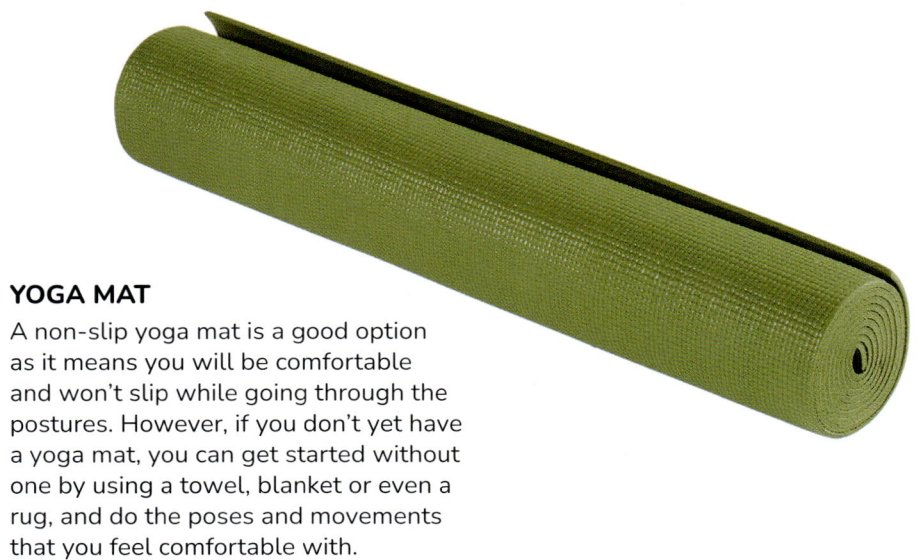

YOGA MAT

A non-slip yoga mat is a good option as it means you will be comfortable and won't slip while going through the postures. However, if you don't yet have a yoga mat, you can get started without one by using a towel, blanket or even a rug, and do the poses and movements that you feel comfortable with.

YOGA BOLSTER

For the relaxation poses and breathing exercises a yoga bolster is useful. I love my bolster and it is also a great support for the deeper poses, like frog (see page 94). It will help to support your body during the restorative or deeper stretches, and enable you to sit upright when you're deep breathing. However, you can also use comfortable sturdier cushions.

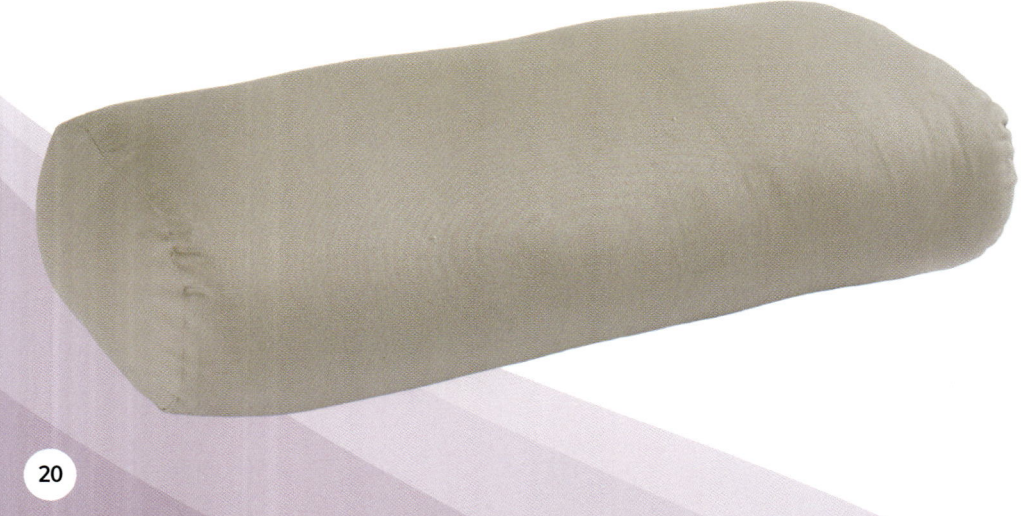

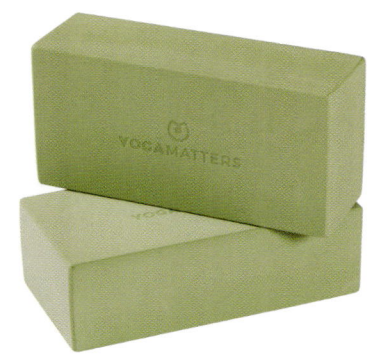

YOGA BRICKS AND BLOCKS

These are great, since they provide support, stability and extension when performing various poses, especially the challenging ones. Equally, you can collect together a few books that are all of a similar size and use those instead.

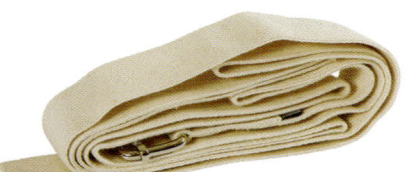

YOGA STRAP

When you're holding poses like the hamstring strap stretch (see page 116), a strap can help you maintain good form and alignment. However, a belt or even a long football sock can be used instead.

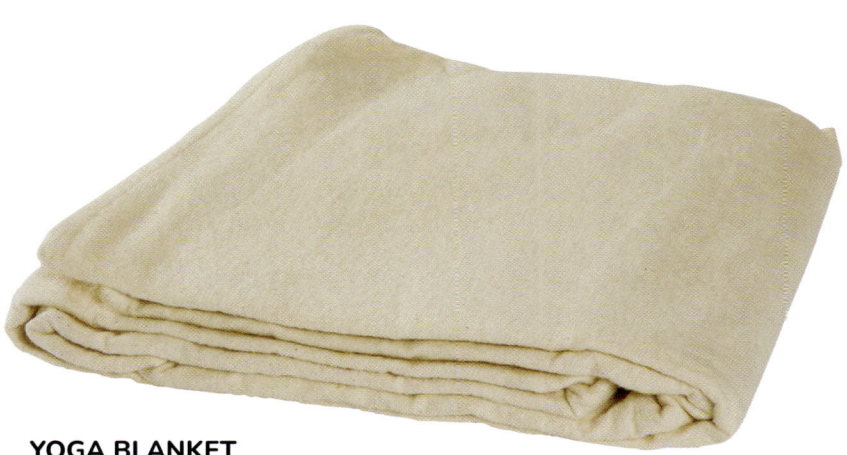

YOGA BLANKET

It's good to be able to slip a blanket under your knees or hips for added padding during certain poses, like pigeon (see page 79). It is also nice to have one to cover yourself with during restorative relaxation poses or when in savasana (see page 72), so you stay warm and cosy. It doesn't have to be a special yoga blanket, though – anything that is fairly soft and can be folded up will work.

5 HOW TO USE THIS BOOK

Whether you're new to yoga or a seasoned practitioner, as someone who plays football – either professionally or for fun – you will find *Yoga for Footballers* is the perfect guide. I have put the specially selected exercises, which I have modified so they deliver exactly what you as a footballer need, into routines.

Part One of the book covers essential daily routines and contains routines for specific times of the day or occasions – morning, pre-training/pre-match, post-training/post-match and evening. Part Two, on the other hand, is called targeted routines and focuses on specific areas of the body – hips, hamstrings, lower back and core. There is also a relaxation routine, including breathing techniques and restorative poses, which are designed to take you to a deeper level of relaxation. The easy-to-follow instructions guide you step by step through the poses, and pictures illustrate the key moments. Some poses have suggested modifications and most have additional notes.

The poses are collated into routines, and it is advisable to start at the beginning, but it is not necessary to always follow through each routine until the end. You can do that if you want to and it feels right, but whether you practise a whole routine in one go or only have time for a couple of exercises, they will still help you feel balanced and healthy. Also, don't feel you need to perfect a pose before moving on – just come back to it another time. Within the routines I have also put together a few flows, which help to take you seamlessly from one pose straight into another.

I recommend you initially take some time to explore the book and familiarise yourself with the various routines, poses, movements and techniques I've included, which are suitable for all players, regardless of your yoga experience or level of football. This will help you select what works best for you, at the right time of day and day of the week, allowing you to tailor your practice to your unique needs and circumstances. Remember, yoga is a personal journey, and every session offers an opportunity to discover something new about yourself.

YOUR JOURNEY WITH FOOTBALL AND YOGA

It may be a cliché, but this practice really is all about the journey and not about reaching a destination. In fact, one of the first things I tell my clients when we practise yoga together is that, unlike football, we are not here to perform. Yoga is about being present in the moment and focusing on the now. You're not here to give 100% as you do in your training sessions or games. Instead, take it slow, listen to your body and be compassionate towards

INTRODUCTION: YOGA AND FOOTBALL

yourself. Ask yourself, 'What do I need today to feel good and be at my best in body, mind and spirit?'

LISTEN TO YOUR BODY

Listening to your body and understanding what it needs every time you practice is crucial to avoiding injury or fatigue. For example, you might intend to complete a full routine, but halfway through, your body may tell you it feels content after just a few poses. It's important to be present, tune in, and notice what your body and mind needs. Adjust accordingly by deciding how many postures, repetitions and sets you want to do today. Tomorrow, or the next day, might feel completely different.

PAUSE FOR THOUGHT

Before you start, take a short moment to reflect on how you're feeling today. Consider factors like how you slept last night, what you ate today or how your training or match went. Was it physically demanding, with any minor injuries, or was it mentally or emotionally exhausting with a lot of pressure? Perhaps it was a late game. This moment of reflection will help you connect with yourself and understand your feelings on a deeper level.

For example, if you've had a mentally demanding game, it might be wise to skip the post-training/post-match routine (see page 58) and focus on the evening routine (see page 74), where slow movements and breathwork will allow for an earlier bedtime. Or if you had an early game, even though you played 90 minutes, you mostly feel the usual post-match fatigue, so it might be beneficial to do both the post-training/post-match routine and focus on the evening routine, as your body and mind will appreciate the extended recovery process these two routines offer.

That is the theory. Now let's get to the practice.

> ## GLOSSARY
>
> **Pose**: Physical postures that promote balance, strength and flexibility.
>
> **Routine (or sequence)**: The way in which yoga poses are placed in a particular order to create a yoga practice with a logical flow or focus on a particular outcome.
>
> **Flow**: This refers to the fluidity of a movement, like a smooth transition from one pose immediately into another, following the breath.

PART ONE

ESSENTIAL DAILY ROUTINES

01 Morning routine ·· page 26
02 Pre-training/pre-match routine ········· page 40
03 Post-training/post-match routine ··· page 58
04 Evening routine ·· page 74

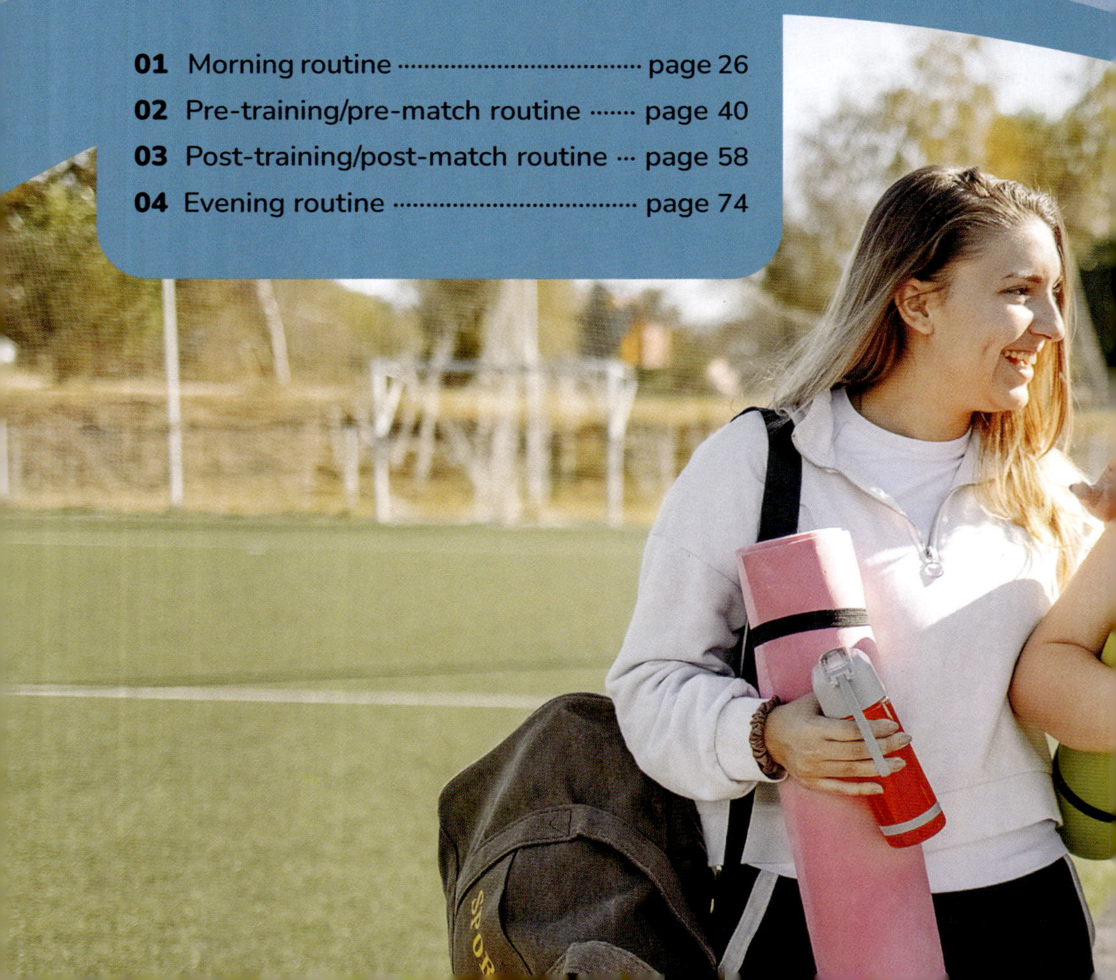

Each one of these four yoga routines has been carefully put together to support different phases of your day, whether it's waking your body up, preparing for high-level performance before training or a match, aiding your recovery afterwards, or winding down at the end of the day.

For the best results, I recommend you incorporate them all into your daily schedule. However, I understand that time can sometimes be limited, so each routine is structured to allow flexibility: for maximum benefit complete the entire sequence, but when time is short focus on the initial segments. The postures are designed to flow seamlessly, enabling you to move smoothly from one pose to the next.

The further you progress into each routine, the more profound the benefits, but even if you can only commit to the first few poses, or just one or two of them, you will still experience significant physical and mental gains. Consistency is key, though, so make these routines a regular part of your day to enhance your performance, recovery and overall wellbeing.

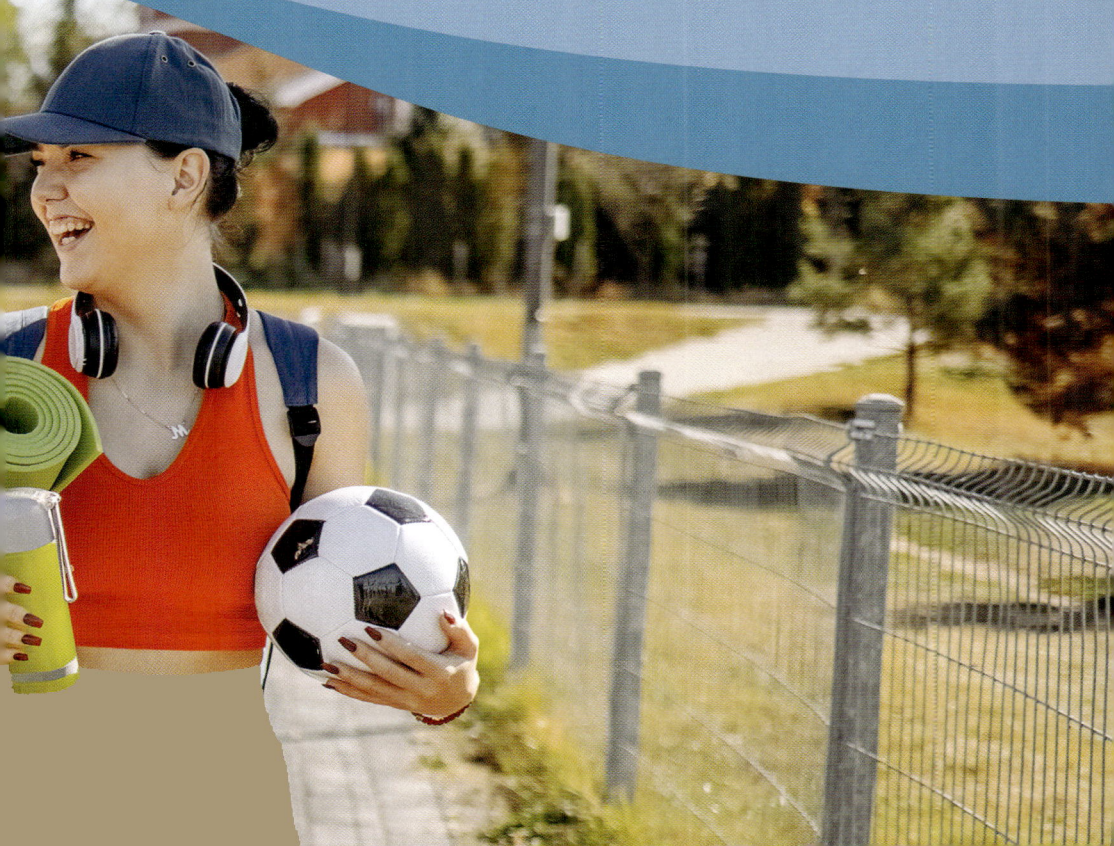

01 MORNING ROUTINE

1 Cat and cow .... page 28
2 Figure of eight .... page 29
3 Standing spinal twist .... page 30
4 Neck stretches .... page 32
5 Rock 'n' rolls .... page 33
6 Sun salutation .... page 34
7 Namaste .... page 36
8 Lunge variations .... page 38
9 Box breathing .... page 39

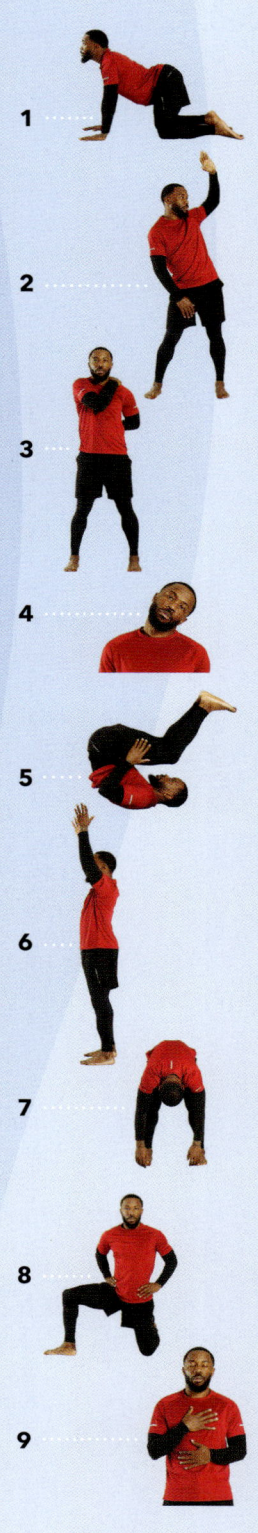

Whatever level you play at, these exercises are ideal for waking up the mind and the body at the start of the day.

Consistency is key for footballers and establishing a morning routine is fundamental for promoting discipline, enhancing performance, and physically and mentally preparing yourself for the demands of the day ahead, on and off the pitch.

The yoga poses and movements in this routine enhance full-body flexibility and mobility, allowing the body to gently open up, increasing new fluid to the joints, supporting cardiovascular circulation, and allowing nutrients and oxygen to be delivered to the muscles by promoting blood flow. The breathwork helps deepen the awakening of body and mind, enhancing the capacity and efficiency of the lungs, and boosting stamina, while activating the parasympathetic nervous system to help you stay calm and focused throughout the day.

The yoga, movement and breathwork in this routine have also been specifically chosen to help facilitate your body's natural detox process by supporting your lymphatic system. Not many people know about this system, but it is a very important one and hence it is vital to support it.

Your body is so intelligent that while you're sleeping your organs digest what you've eaten across the day, repair the tissue you damaged during training and eliminate the toxins that have built up. The lymphatic system flushes out this accumulated waste, but it relies on gentle movement, muscle contractions and deep breathing to kickstart it.

Keeping your lymphatic system functioning effectively will not only help you digest your food better, and reduce the inflammation caused by everyday training, but it also supports your performance on the pitch, keeping your energy levels high throughout the day, and boosting your immune system and thus your overall wellbeing.

LEMON WATER

Although it is not specifically yoga related, starting your day with a cup of lemon water is a refreshing and rejuvenating way to hydrate your body. Unlike plain water, freshly squeezed lemon juice is a natural source of vital nutrients like vitamins C and B, as well as minerals such as calcium and magnesium. Among many other benefits it boosts the immune system, balances body pH and promotes digestive health.

One of the most important reasons why I recommend lemon water first thing in the morning is that it supports the lymphatic system and assists in detoxification by encouraging the liver to flush out the toxins built up overnight.

To rejuvenate your mind and deeply hydrate and energise your body for the day ahead, squeeze half a lemon (or lime) into a large glass (at least 450ml or 16 fl oz) of purified, room-temperature water and drink.

Lemon water is also an ideal pre- and post-training drink, so you can make up a big jug and drink it throughout the day to continue to cleanse and hydrate your body.

1 CAT AND COW

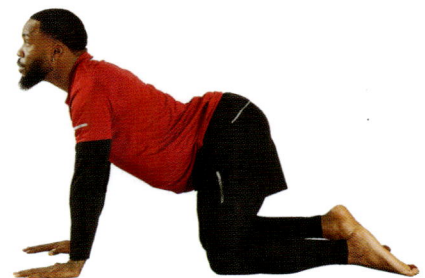 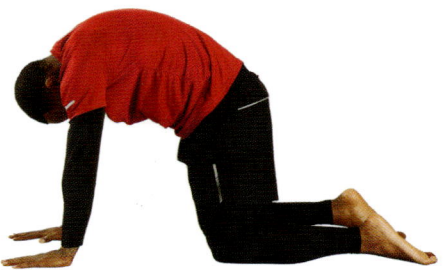

Cat and cow is great as a warm-up on its own or as a part of the beginning of any programme. I have included it here as part of your morning routine since it is great for stretching and mobilising the spine, creating space in between the vertebrates and surrounding areas, improving flexibility and blood circulation in the body.

This flow of movement primarily supports a greater range of motion and spinal health by enhancing the flexibility and mobility of your spine, and indirectly also promoting better hip mobility. It is a great way to boost your energy levels and to awaken the body first thing in the morning. What is even more effective while in this flow is to focus on deep breaths and synchronise it with each movement. This will accelerate your blood flow and improve circulation around the body, but specially around the spine which will in turn support the lymphatic system in flushing out waste and toxins.

Other benefits of focusing on the breath while flowing through this movement, and particularly first thing in the morning, is it will give you a meditative moment which will help you to enhance the connection with yourself and to align with your intentions for your day, whether you have a training session ahead or a game.

1. Begin on your hands and knees, in a tabletop position. Make sure your wrists, elbows and shoulders are in line, your knees are below your hips, hip-width apart, and your spine is in a neutral position, neither arched nor rounded.

2. As you inhale, drop your belly down, lift your head and chest up, and move your shoulders away from your ears (cow).

3. As you exhale, round your spine gently, bringing your chin towards your chest, as far as it feels comfortable (cat).

4. Move with a smooth flow between the cat and cow poses, allowing the length of your breath to be the length of each pose.

5. Repeat this flow of movement for several breaths, focusing on your breath and the movement of your spine. Imagine each vertebrae moves one at a time, starting from your tail bone and hips, then moving up through your lower back, mid-back, neck and lastly your head.

2 FIGURE OF EIGHT

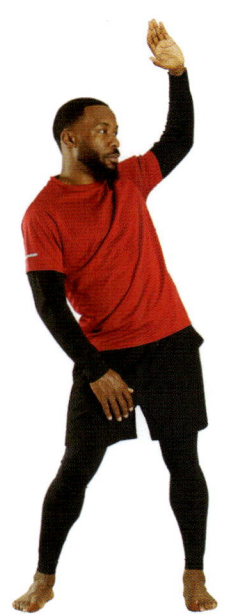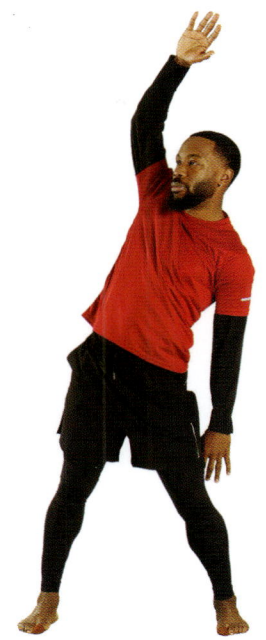

Figure of eight is a great movement for first thing in the morning. It stimulates blood flow, and awakens the mind and body, loosening muscles stiff from the hours in bed. The increase in blood flow can also boost energy levels and create mental sharpness.

It supports an increase in range of motion by engaging the shoulders, hip joints and deep core. The activation of these important muscles enhances stability and power, and sets you up for your day ahead.

1. Stand upright with your feet shoulder-width apart.

2. As you inhale, start moving your hips to the right to begin making a (sideways) figure of eight.

3. As you exhale, shift your weight and your hips to the left.

4. Inhale and move your hips back to the right again.

5. When you find a nice flow, incorporate your arms as well – as you move your hips to the right, move your arms to the right, and so on.

6. Continue for a couple of minutes, until you feel warm and loosened up.

7. Once you feel comfortable, you can spread your feet further apart. As you move from side to side, you will start feeling it in your groin muscles. That makes this a great groin-lengthening exercise too, so it is also very good for a pre- or post-training or match routine.

3 STANDING SPINAL TWIST

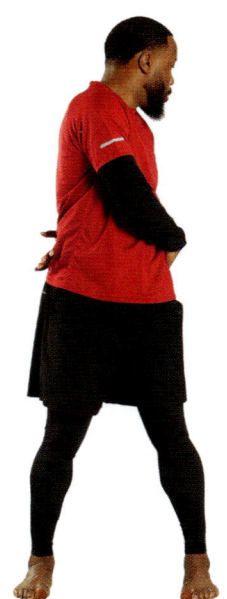
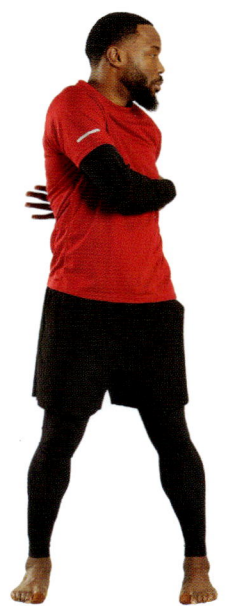
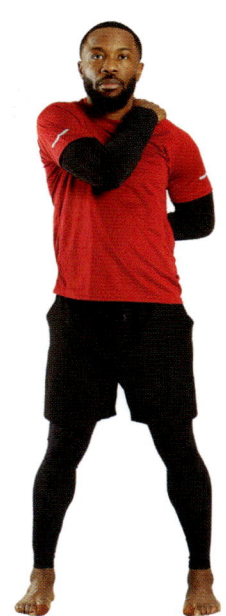

Including the standing spinal twist in your morning routine can be particularly beneficial as it helps to awaken the body in many ways. As you do the twist movements, blood flow increases, and flexibility and mobility in the joints and muscles of the spine, hips, shoulders and arms improve.

What I also love about this twist is that not only does it support you from a flexibility, mobility and stability perspective, when you tap around the back of the hips and lower back, it also stimulates the kidneys and promotes good kidney function. This is essential for filtering waste from the blood and stimulates the lymphatic system, which helps remove metabolic waste and toxins, leading to increased vitality, mental clarity and overall wellbeing.

1. Stand with your feet hip-width apart, or wider, a slight softness in your knees and arms at your sides.

2. Inhale and as you exhale gently twist your body to your right, then back to the centre and then to your left, initiating the movement from the lower part of your spine. Each time you twist, look over your shoulder or behind you if you can.

3. Find a natural rhythm to the twisting movement, allowing your arms to swing, and gently tap your hands on your lower back and hip area.

4. Breathing slowly and deeply, continue the twists and move up to your mid-back, moving your arms and gently tapping in your thoracic area.

5. Steadily moving further up your upper back, allow one arm to go behind you and tap in your shoulder blade area, and your other arm to cross your chest and tap your upper shoulder muscles.

6. In your own time slowly reverse the twist and work your way back down, stopping at your mid-back area before finishing at your lower spine.

7. If you have time, do another one or two rounds, thinking about your breath as you move through, inhaling in the centre and exhaling as you twist.

ADD IN MUSCLE MASSAGE

When you're twisting the upper part of your body and tapping your upper shoulder muscles, it can be quite nice to pause and gently dig your fingers into those muscles to massage them. Use your index, middle and ring fingers together and apply gentle pressure in small circular movements, while breathing deeply, for a few minutes or longer if it feels good.

Often these muscles are tight and not only does this limit the range of movement and lead to pain and discomfort in the neck area, but this muscular tightness can also compress blood vessels, which reduces the blood flow to the brain and can lead to headaches, fatigue and decreased cognitive function.

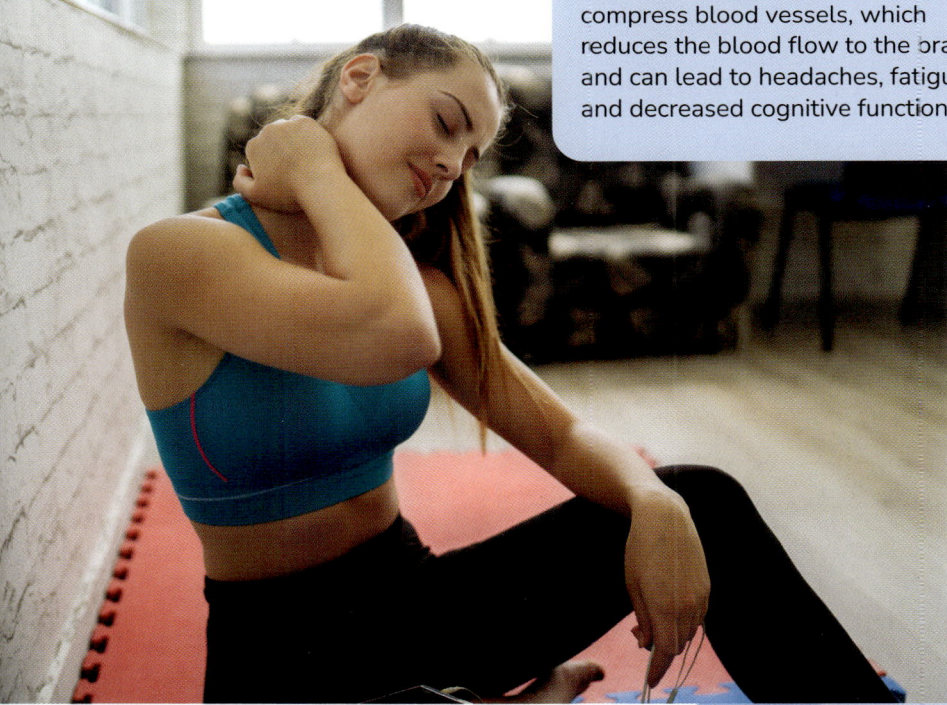

4 NECK STRETCHES

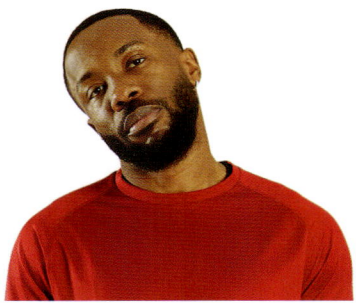
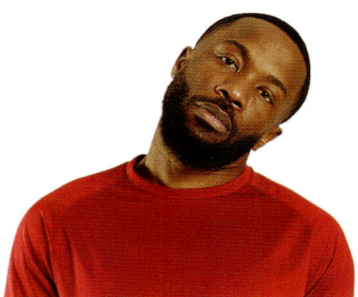
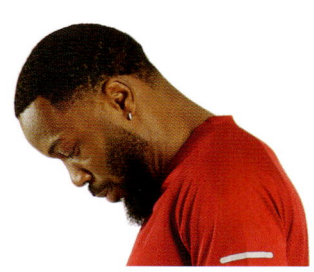
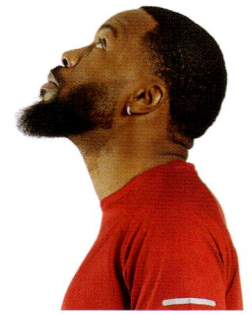

After you have massaged your upper shoulder muscles, you can also add some gentle neck stretches to alleviate tension and improve neck flexibility.

1. Slowly tilt your right ear towards your right shoulder, without lifting your left shoulder. Hold this position for 10 to 15 seconds, breathing deeply and slowly throughout, before slowly switching sides. Repeat for two to three rounds or until you feel the tension has released.

2. Slowly move your chin down towards your chest, pausing for a breath or two, before gently moving your head up and back (not all the way back) and looking up towards the ceiling. Repeat two to three times, or more if that feels good, breathing deeply and slowly throughout.

5 ROCK 'N' ROLLS

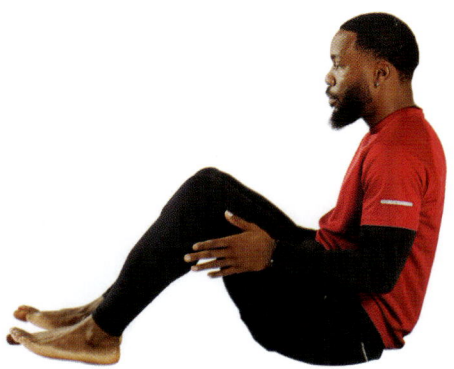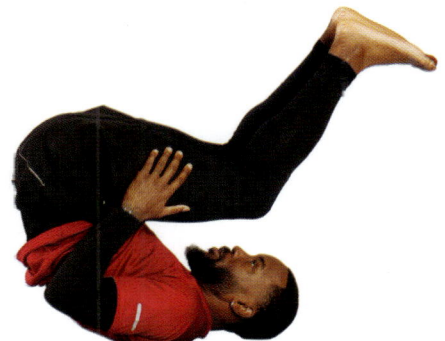

Rock 'n' rolls is a great movement to incorporate into your morning routine. It's ideal for starting your day as it helps to release stiffness and tension in the spine, particularly in the lower back area. The forward and backward rolling action stimulates circulation and gently massages the spinal muscles, enhancing both flexibility and mobility. Adding this exercise to your morning routine can help you wake up your body and prepare it for the day ahead.

1. Sit with your knees bent and your feet on the floor, keeping your hands gently on your legs, just below your knees.

2. Inhale and as you exhale rock backwards on to your back, lifting your feet and legs off the floor, and allowing your legs to move freely and as far or little back as feels natural.

3. On the same exhale, rock forwards by gently pressing your hands into your legs, and come on to your sit bones and initial position, keeping your spine nice and long.

4. Continue to rock backwards and forwards, allowing your breath to lead the movements, for as many times as it feels good.

6 SUN SALUTATION

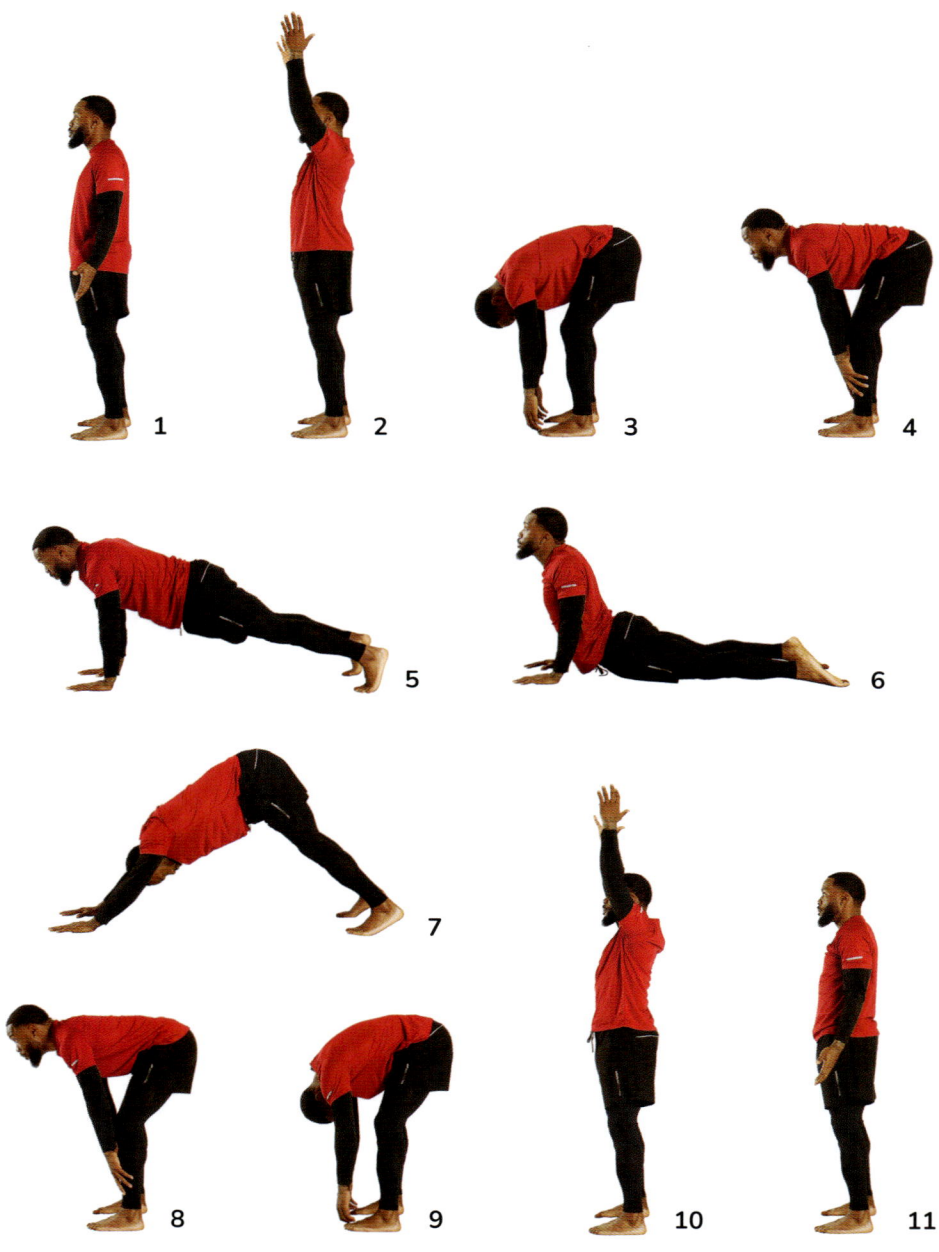

01 MORNING ROUTINE

Sun salutation offers great benefits for footballers because it activates the major muscle groups, joints and soft tissue. Coordinating breath with movement is also a great way of waking up the physical body and encouraging mental focus, while providing a natural energy boost.

Sun salutation is an excellent dynamic morning routine by itself or as a warm-up at the start of a flow. In fact, it's a perfect flow to use as a part of your pre–training or pre-match programme, since it prepares the body for the demands of a session or game.

1. Stand tall with your feet hip-width apart, arms relaxed at your sides and palms facing forward.

2. Inhale and raise your arms overhead, face your palms together and gently arch your back.

3. As you exhale, hinge at the hips and fold forward, bringing your hands to the floor beside your feet.

4. Inhale, lengthen your spine and lift your gaze, looking forward and placing your hands on your shins or thighs. Make sure you keep your back flat.

5. As you exhale, step or jump back into a plank position, keeping your arms straight, with your wrists directly under your shoulders so you form a straight line from your head to your heels.

6. Lower your body halfway down, keeping your elbows close to your ribs. Inhale, straighten your arms and lift your chest, keeping your legs and hips off the ground.

7. As you exhale, lift your hips up and back, forming a pyramid shape with your body, pressing your heels towards the floor.

8. Inhale and step or jump your feet to the top of your mat. Lengthen your spine and lift your gaze, looking forward and placing your hands on your shins or thighs, keeping your back flat.

9. As you exhale, fold forward over your legs.

10. Inhale and sweep your arms out to the sides and up overhead as you come up to standing, arching your back slightly.

11. As you exhale, bring your arms back down by your sides, finishing this round.

12. Repeat this sequence as many times as it feels good and your body feels loosened, your mind is sharpened, your breath is moving easily and you are energised.

7 NAMASTE

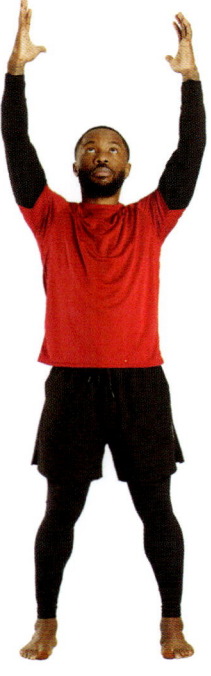
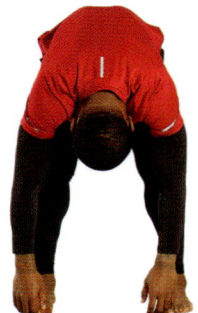
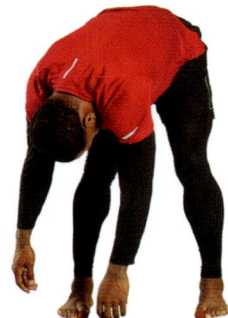

This is one of my favourite movements and one that I always include in all my clients' programmes, regardless of the routine or where they are in their training week. It definitely has an amazing effect if you perform it in the morning.

It opens up the front, side and back line of the body, helping to reduce stiffness in all those areas. As you open up the chest and arms, and reach up overhead, you will stretch the shoulders and upper back, increasing mobility in those areas. Then, as you fold forward you will feel tension in the spine and tightness in the back, especially the lower back, being released. If your calves and hamstrings are tight you will feel them, too, being stretched as you fold forward.

This full movement releases stress, anxiety and fatigue, so while in the forward bend you will feel a sense of calm and tranquillity, but at the same time you will feel rejuvenated due to the increase of oxygen to your muscles and organs.

1. Stand with your feet hip-width apart and your arms at your sides. Be aware of your posture, stand tall and tuck your shoulder blades in slightly.

2. As you inhale, open up your chest and lift your arms up towards the ceiling, gently arching your back as you look up towards your hands. These can be facing each other or your palms can be touching.

3. As you exhale, bring your hands down through the midline of your body and, with your chin tucked in to your chest, slowly move them towards the floor and bend forwards.

4. Releasing your hands, allow your fingers to touch the floor. If your fingers don't touch the floor, bend your knees slightly. You might also need to bend your knees if your hamstrings are very tight, but if so, do make sure your hips are still as high as possible.

5. Bend forward, with at least your fingertips touching the floor and your head heavy.

6. Move your hips from side to side, allowing your fingers to draw semi-circles, for a breath or two.

7. When you feel ready to come up, keep your chin near your chest and slowly roll up, with your head coming up last. As you open your chest, lift your arms up towards the sky and look up towards your hands again. That is one round.

8. Continue this flow for five to six rounds or until you feel loosened up, making sure you breathe deeply throughout the movement.

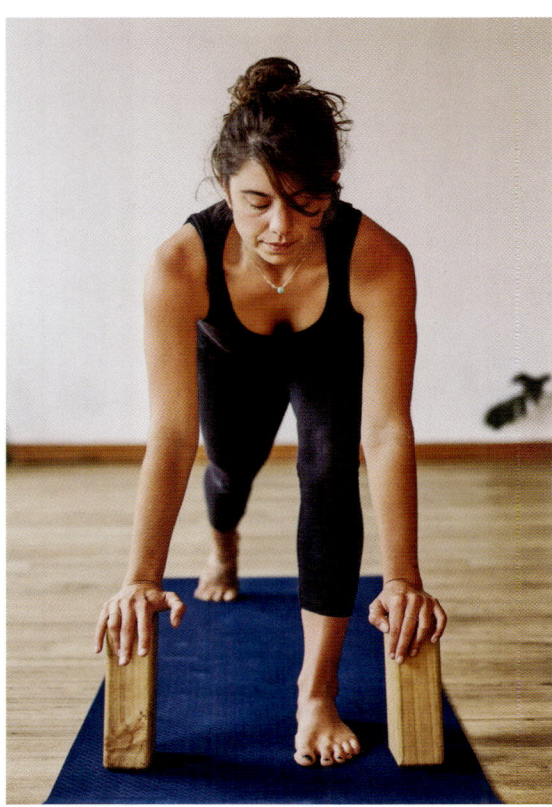

YOGA FOR FOOTBALLERS

8 LUNGE VARIATIONS

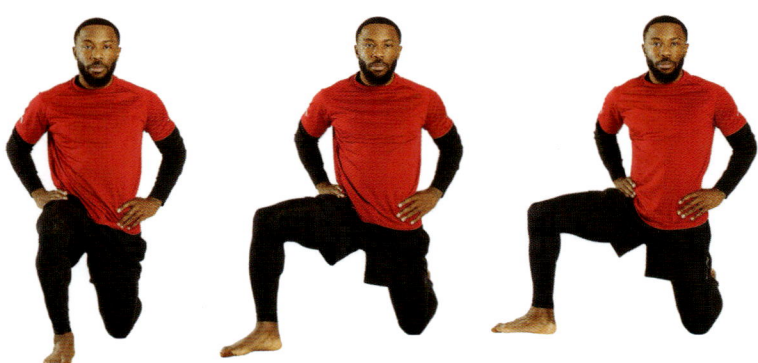

As a footballer you rely on the mobility of your hips, particularly when sprinting, changing direction and, of course, kicking. This variation on the lunge helps open up the hip flexors and groin muscles, and hence when practised regularly it gives a greater range of motion in the hip joint.

Moving into the different positions needed for this lunge requires balance and that strengthens the stabilising muscles of the ankles, knees and hips. This stability, also called proprioception, is essential for footballers as it helps you sense your body position and coordinate movements, especially complex ones, like dribbling and passing.

With increased flexibility, this pose will also help you reduce the risk of common football injuries.

1. Start in a lunge position with your left knee and shin on the floor, and your right leg forward with your foot on the floor, and ankle and knee in a line, as if your front foot is in the 12 o'clock position on a clock face.

2. Engage your core muscles by gently squeezing your belly button towards your spine. Keep your shoulders and hips stacked and inline, your spine nice and long, and your tail bone (the base of your spine) pointing down towards the floor, so your hips are in neutral and not tilting. Place your hands on your hips.

3. Inhale and as you exhale move your right leg and place your foot at 2 o'clock. Notice the difference in this position compared to the previous one.

4. On your next exhale, move your right leg and foot to 3 o'clock. Notice how the stretch changes and where you now feel it.

5. Inhale and as you exhale come all the way back to 12 o'clock with your right leg and foot.

6. Slowly bring your left leg forward and switch sides.

7. From 12 o'clock move to 10 o'clock and then 9 o'clock before coming back to 12 o'clock.

8. Do this sequence two to three times on each side, focusing on slow, deep breaths. The length of your breath can be the length of the movement or you can move at a slower pace if that feels better.

01 MORNING ROUTINE

9 BOX BREATHING

BOX BREATHING

Integrating breathwork into your morning routine will optimise your performance, enhance your recovery and promote your overall wellbeing. Box breathing is a simple yet very powerful breathwork technique, which supports the flow of blood and oxygen to your muscles and your brain.

Find a relaxed position, either lying down or sitting comfortably with your spine straight. Take a couple of normal breaths before you begin.

When you are ready, slowly breathe in through your nose, keeping your mouth closed, for a count of four.

Once you have fully inhaled, hold your breath for four counts, making sure you're not tensing your body and are in a relaxed state.

Gently breathe out through your nose, or mouth, whatever feels good, for a count of four, and notice how the air is released from your body.

Once you have exhaled, hold your breath again for a count of four. You have now finished the cycle and completed one round.

Continue the cycle for four rounds or as many as feels comfortable, but it's good to gradually increase your practice over time.

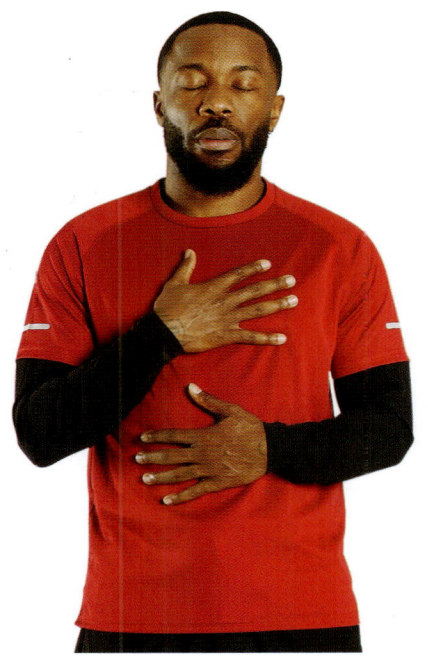

NOTE

Box breathing is usually considered safe for most people. However, since it involves holding your breath, it is not recommended for people with high blood pressure or those with heart, lung, ear or eye issues. For the same reason, it is also not recommended for pregnant women or those with severe anxiety or other medical conditions, such as epilepsy or vertigo. If you have any of these conditions or any health concerns, speak to your doctor or health care provider before doing box breathing or any of the breath techniques in this book. Even if you're not in any of the risk groups, if you feel dizzy or experience any type of discomfort while performing this breathing technique, you should stop and resume normal breathing.

02 PRE-TRAINING/ PRE-MATCH ROUTINE

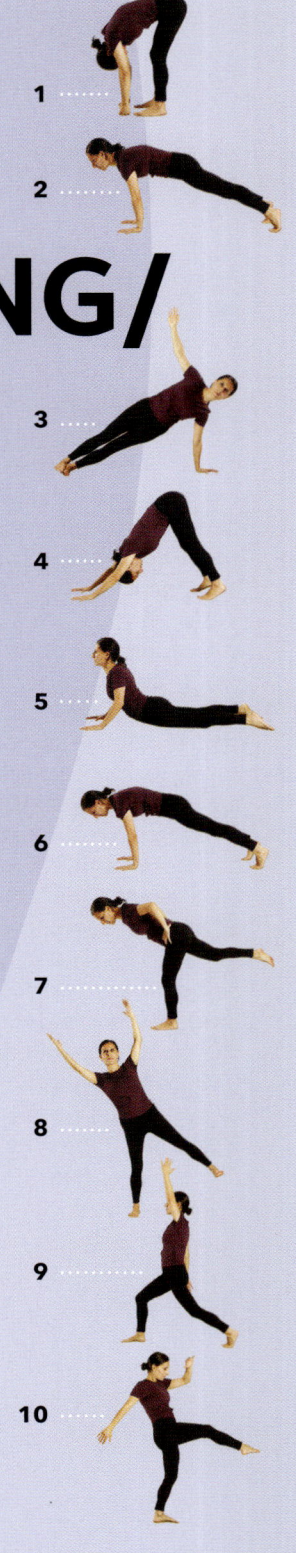

1 Namaste .... page 42
2 Yoga plank .... page 44
3 Yoga side plank .... page 46
4 Downward-facing dog .... page 48
5 Cobra .... page 50
6 Downward-facing dog to cobra .... page 51
7 Warrior 3 .... page 53
8 Football star .... page 54
9 High lunge flow .... page 55
10 Football yoga flow .... page 57

Yoga can be an incredibly beneficial way of preparing the body and mind before a training session or a game.

02 PRE-TRAINING/PRE-MATCH ROUTINE

In this section I have chosen poses and flows that will set you up both mentally and physically for the training session or game ahead, preparing you for the physical and mental demands of training or competition, and allowing your body to warm up properly.

They will also help strengthen, stabilise and activate the muscles, which in return will improve your stamina, balance and coordination, but when practising them you also need to pay attention to your breath and being 'in the now'. Think about your alignment and any sensations you feel in your body because this will allow you to stay present, improve your concentration and therefore reduce the risk of injuries.

As well as enhancing your overall performance on the pitch, these poses and flows will help give you a sense of calmness and clarity. You will feel ready to take on all the demands of your training session or game, setting yourself up for success.

You can add as many of these exercises as you wish into the preparation you're doing already. Choose a few of the poses, or a flow, or do them all back-to-back, in order, as I have made sure you can move easily from one to another.

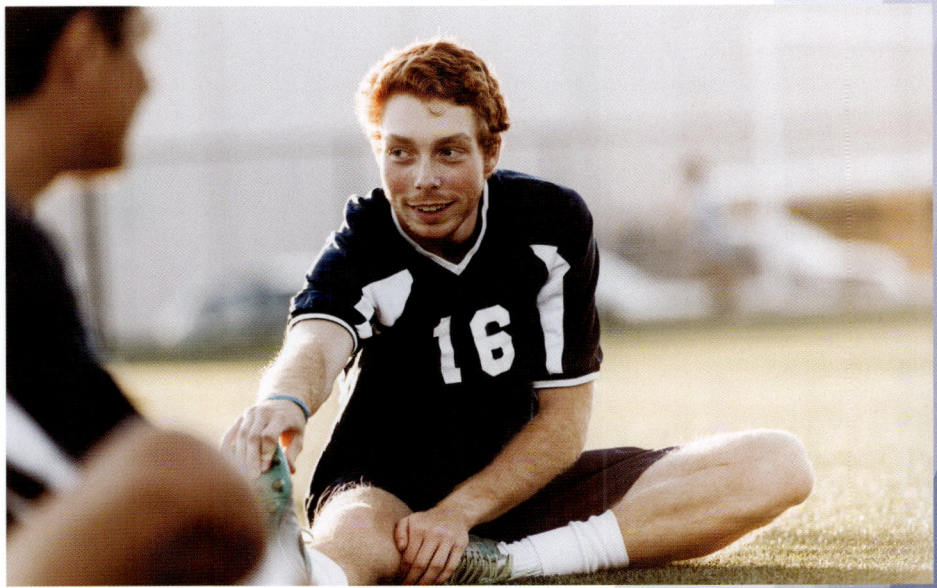

1 NAMASTE

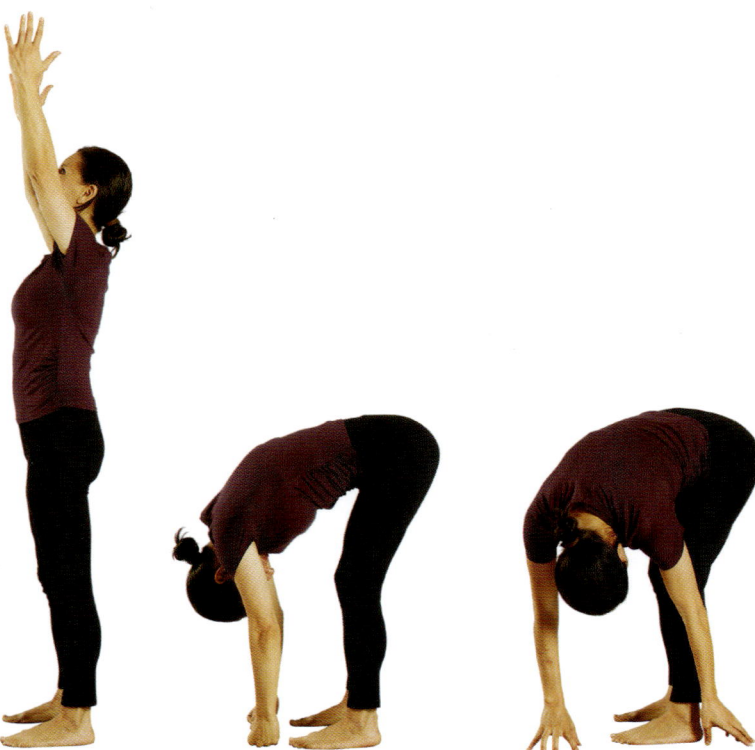

You'll recognise this movement from the morning routine (see page 36). As I've said, it is one of my favourites and I always incorporate it into my clients' programmes, regardless of their routine or training schedule. I call it 'namaste' because every time my clients come up to a standing position and place their palms together, we say 'namaste'.

This movement is excellent for opening up the front, side and back lines of the body, helping to increase flexibility. As you open your chest and extend your arms overhead, you'll stretch your shoulders and upper back, again, improving your flexibility. When you fold forward, you'll feel tension in your spine and lower back release. If your calves and hamstrings are tight, you'll also experience a stretch in those areas as you bend forward.

In this position, touching the floor and with your head below your heart, the increased blood flow to your brain helps to sharpen focus, preparing you for the coming exertions. As you sway from side to side, you'll feel your side body and hips opening up, enhancing flexibility in these areas. This movement helps to release any lingering tension, ensuring your body is fully warmed up and ready for what is ahead.

1. Stand with your feet hip-width apart and your arms at your sides. Be aware of your posture, stand tall and tuck your shoulder blades in slightly.

2. As you inhale, open up your chest and lift your arms up towards the ceiling, gently arching your back as you look up towards your hands. These can be facing each other or your palms can be touching.

3. As you exhale, bring your hands down through the midline of your body and, with your chin tucked in to your chest, slowly move them towards the floor and bend forwards.

4. Releasing your hands, allow your fingers to touch the floor. If your fingers don't touch the floor, bend your knees slightly. You might also need to bend your knees if your hamstrings are very tight, but if so, do make sure your hips are still as high as possible.

5. Bend forward, with at least your fingertips touching the floor and your head heavy.

6. Move your hips from side to side, allowing your fingers to draw semi-circles, for a breath or two.

7. When you feel ready to come up, keep your chin near your chest and slowly roll up, with your head coming up last. As you open your chest, lift your arms up towards the sky and look up towards your hands again. That is one round.

8. Continue this flow for five to six rounds or until you feel loosened up, making sure you breathe deeply throughout the movement.

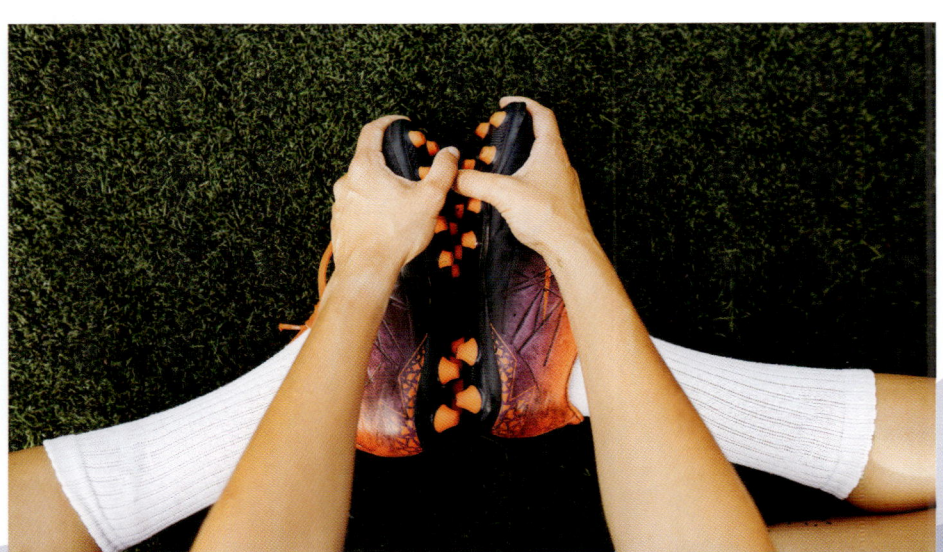

2 YOGA PLANK

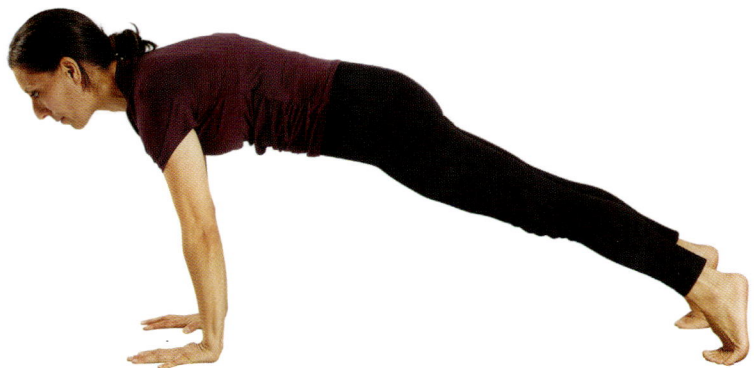

In yoga, we hold the plank with the arms straight, rather than the traditional plank performed with the forearms down. Although both are similar, the yoga plank engages a wider range of muscle groups simultaneously, allowing the upper body muscles to be included more effectively, while restoring healthier spinal and pelvic alignment. That is why this version is more suitable for footballers.

The yoga plank strengthens the entire core, including the deep stabilising muscles, as well as the glutes, muscles of the upper back, chest, shoulders, arms and wrists. It increases stability and balance, especially in the shoulders and hips, which are crucial for maintaining control and power during dynamic movements on the pitch.

1. Begin on your hands and knees, in a tabletop position. Make sure your wrists, elbows and shoulders are in line, your knees are below your hips, hip-width apart, and your spine is in a neutral position, neither arched nor rounded.

2. Inhale and as you exhale extend your legs one at a time behind you. Keep your body and legs straight, from your head all the way to your heels, with your heels above and in line with the base of your toes.

3. Activate your core muscles by imagining you're lifting your belly button up and in towards your spine.

4. Make sure your hands and arms are shoulder-width apart, and then gently shift your weight forward, allowing your shoulders to be slightly over your wrists.

02 PRE-TRAINING/PRE-MATCH ROUTINE

5. Keeping your neck and head in line with your spine, and your gaze soft, looking slightly in front of you, focus on your breath, breathing deeply and slowly, in and out.

6. Hold this pose for 30 seconds, or longer if it's comfortable, but your alignment is key here, so it is advisable to gradually increase the duration over time.

7. When you're ready to come out of the pose (if you're not flowing in to another one), gently lower your knees back down to the floor.

NOTE
If you do have wrist injuries, then it is advisable to do the plank on the forearms or to skip this pose.

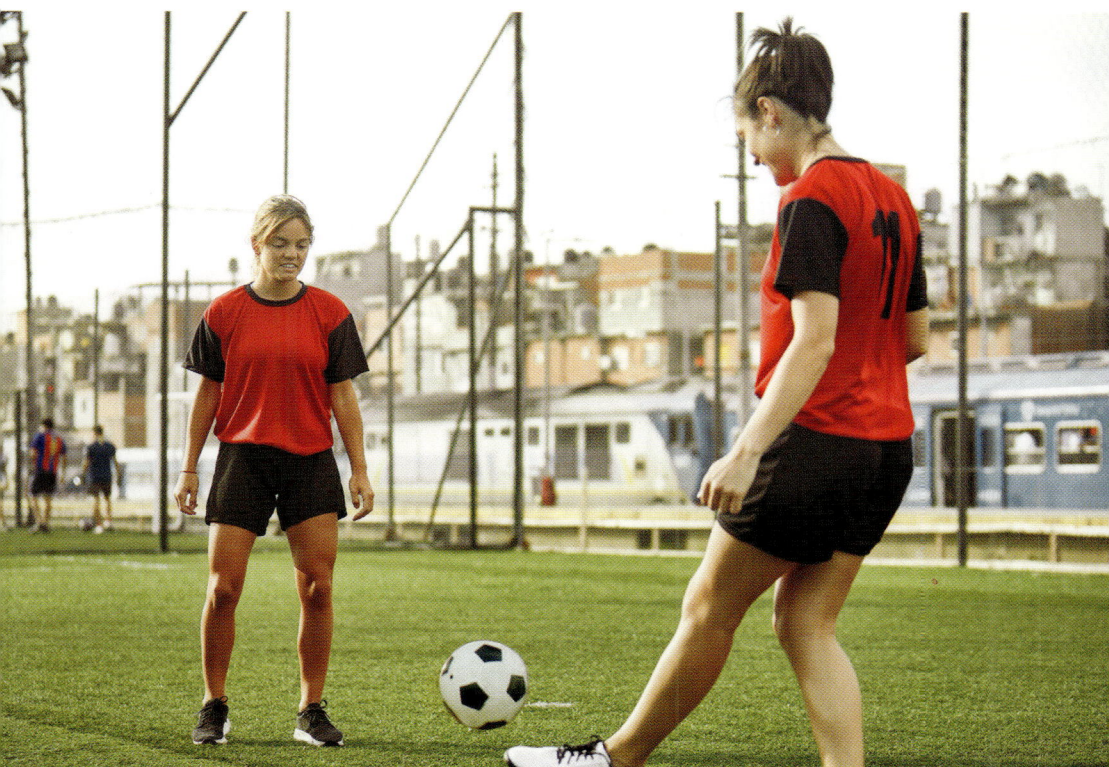

3 YOGA SIDE PLANK

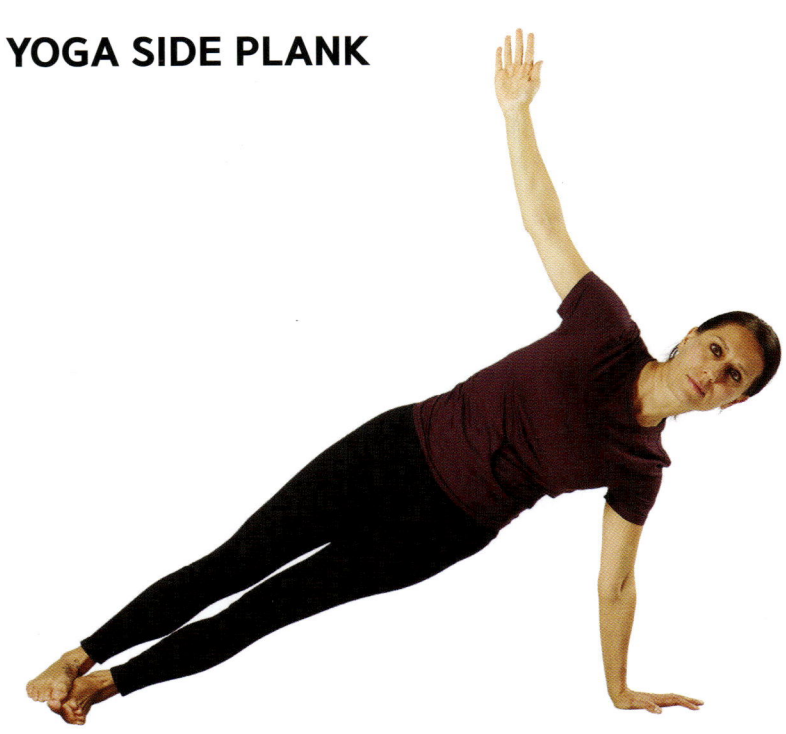

Like the yoga plank, the yoga side plank works on the core and upper body, improving strength, stability, posture, balance and coordination. And just like the yoga plank, as a part of a pre-training or pre-match routine, it helps reduce the risk of injury, enhances performance and sharpens mental focus. When practised regularly it improves posture and good alignment of the pelvis and spine.

Since the arm is straight here, rather than the forearm being on the floor, as in the traditional side plank, it helps strengthen the upper back, shoulder and arm muscles, while improving the stability, balance and control on the side of the body that is closest to the floor.

This side body position, with the arm straight out, mimics a football-specific move, when one player holds another player off by extending their arm, so that they can then, for example, pass the ball.

1. Start in a yoga plank (see page 44), keeping a straight line from the top of your head to your heels, with your wrists, elbows and shoulders aligned.

2. Move your weight on to your left hand and the edge of your left foot. From here, you can either stack your right foot on top of the left one or place it on the floor slightly in front of the left, which will give you more stability.

3. Inhale and as you exhale gently lift yourself up, making sure your hips are lifted and in line with your shoulder and your left wrist, elbow and shoulder are aligned.

4. Move your right arm up towards the ceiling so that it forms a straight line with your shoulders.

5. Hold this pose for 15 to 30 seconds, or longer if it feels comfortable and you're in good alignment.

6. Focus on your breath, breathing deeply and slowly, in and out.

7. When you're ready to release, bring your right arm back down on to the floor, so you come into a plank. Then switch on to your right arm and repeat on the other side.

MODIFIED YOGA SIDE PLANK

A great variation for beginners or those who are coming back from an injury and have restricted mobility and/or strength, a modified yoga side plank is performed just like the side plank, with the left hand on the floor and the left arm straight, with the right arm straight up in the air, and the shoulders stacked. The difference, though, is that the left knee is bent and rests on the ground, which keeps the pelvis and hips more stable. Don't forget to repeat on the other side.

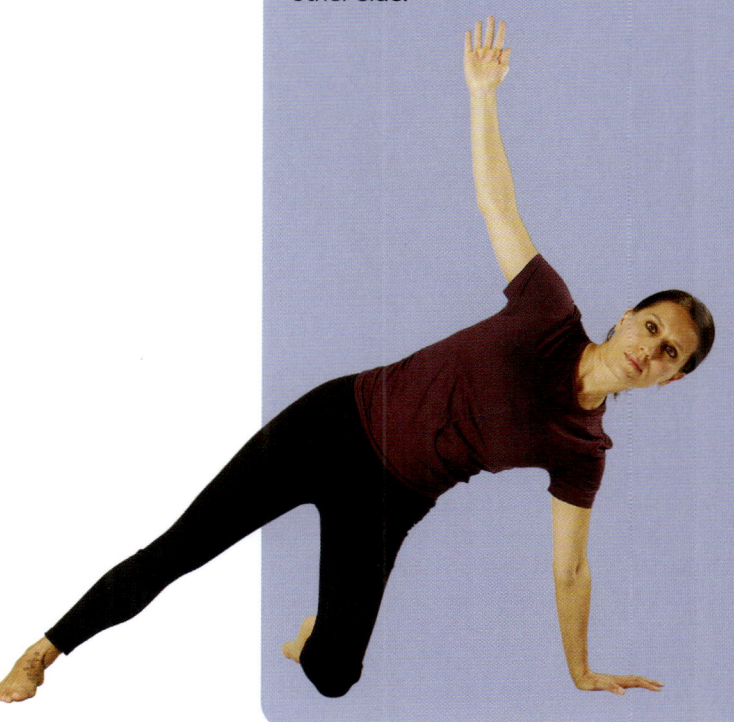

4 DOWNWARD-FACING DOG

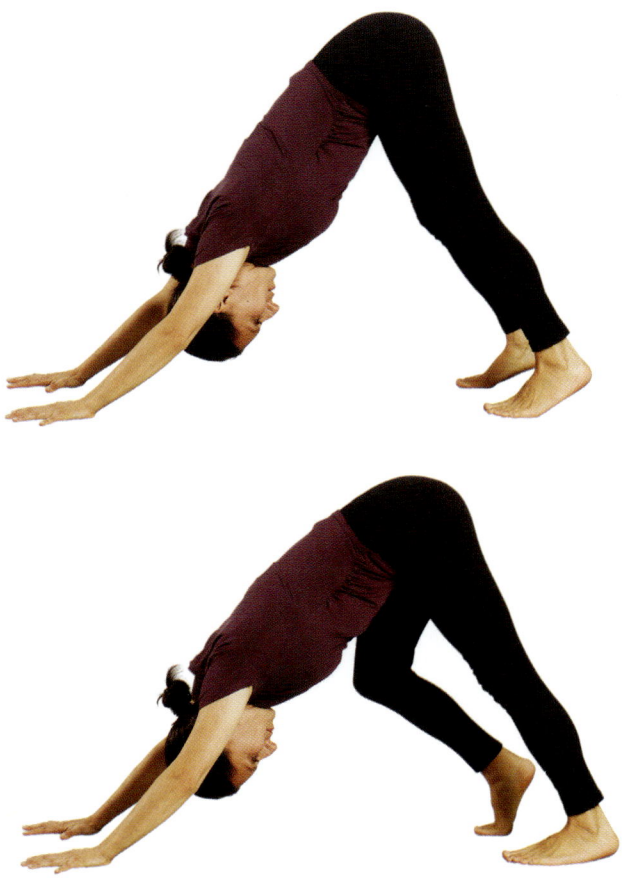

The downward-facing dog is another of those amazing poses that I highly recommend players perform every day and as a part of any routine. I have included it in the pre-training/pre-match routine because it is a great way of warming up the body. Since you're in an inverted position, with your head below your heart, the blood flow to the head is stimulated, leaving you feeling energised, rejuvenated and focused for your game or training session ahead.

The downward-facing dog lengthens the whole of the back of the body, which improves flexibility and hence helps reduce the risk of injuries. It also strengthens the upper body and leg muscles, and activates the core too, so can therefore increase physical performance. It can be done by itself, or it goes well as a flow together with the yoga plank (see page 44) and cobra (see page 50).

1. Begin on your hands and knees, in a tabletop position. Make sure your wrists are slightly in front of your shoulders, and your knees are below your hips, hip-width apart.

2. Inhale fully and as you exhale lift your hips high up, imagining your tail bone is pointing up towards the ceiling. Bend your knees slightly or as much as is necessary to keep your hips up high.

3. Continue to inhale and exhale as you keep your spine straight, your chest close to the front of your thighs, your arms straight, and your shoulder blades slightly down (away from your ears) and tucked in. Your feet should be parallel, hip-width apart, or slightly wider if that feels better for you, and your palms should be fully pressed down, with your fingers spread wide.

4. Keep your neck and head relaxed, gaze towards your belly button and gently draw your belly button towards your spine to activate your core muscles.

5. Focus on all these points and take deep, slow breaths.

6. Start 'pedalling' your feet, gently moving your heels towards the floor one at a time. You can also combine the 'pedalling' with short holds, for 15 seconds or so, and then go back to pedalling again.

7. Slowly bring your knees down to the floor (shake your wrists out if you want to), then go back up and repeat a couple of times.

NOTE
Your heels don't have to touch the floor and, if your chest and shoulders are very tight, your hands can be slightly wider apart.

If your shoulders and chest are very tight, practise the cobra (see page 50) before the downward-facing dog, as it will help open up those areas and make the downward-facing dog easier.

5 COBRA

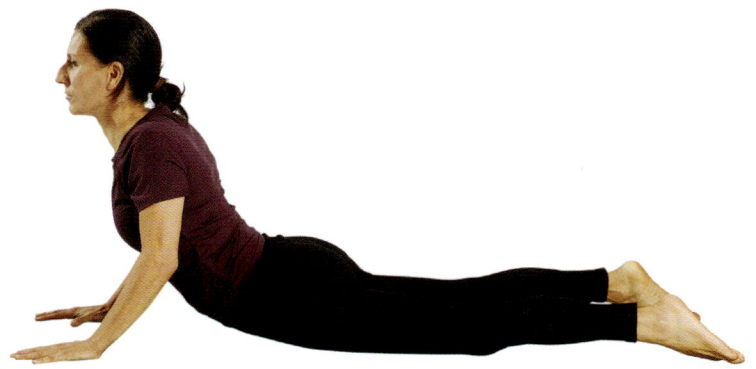

As a player you tend to make a lot of repetitive movements and this often places a strain on your back, but the cobra is very beneficial for footballers because it's great for spinal health. This pose brings a rich supply of blood to your back, increasing the flexibility and mobility of the spine. In fact, it strengthens the core, glutes and muscles of the whole back, as well as opening the front of the body and stretching out the chest and shoulders. When practised regularly, it significantly improves posture.

1. Lie flat on your front, with your legs extended and the front of your ankles on the floor. Your feet can be apart or your big toes can be touching.

2. Place your palms on the floor, directly under your shoulders, making sure your fingers are pointing forwards and are wide apart.

3. Inhale and as you exhale press your hands on to the floor while gently lifting your chest and upper body away from it. Keep your lower abdomen on the floor.

4. Tuck your elbows in to your body and relax your shoulders.

5. Focus on the pose by opening your chest forward and upward, keeping your gaze forwards or ever so slightly upwards.

6. Hold the pose for 15 to 30 seconds, while breathing deeply and slowly.

7. Come out of the pose on an exhale, and slowly lower your chest and upper body down.

8. Once you release the pose, roll your hips from side to side, which will feel nice in your lower back.

NOTE
In general, you should not feel any pain in your lower back while in this pose. However, if you feel pressure in your lower back or in the front of your hip bones, place a folded blanket in front of your hips. If you feel any pinching or pain in your lower back, widen the distance between your feet, which will create more space for your hips and pelvis.

02 PRE-TRAINING/PRE-MATCH ROUTINE

6 DOWNWARD-FACING DOG TO COBRA

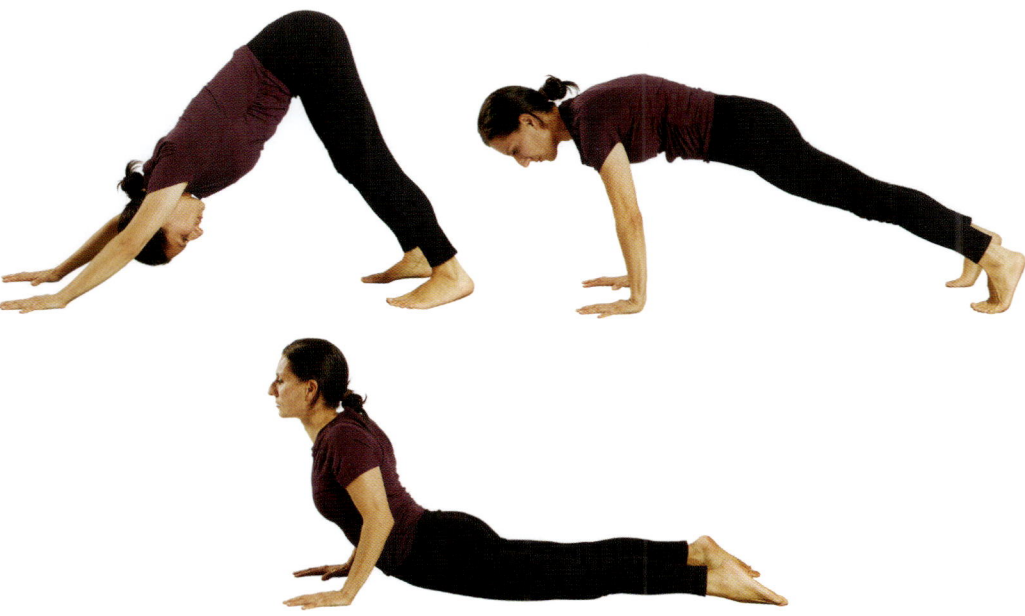

This flow – from downward-facing dog to cobra – works on strength, stability, flexibility and mobility. In downward-facing dog you stretch from the back of your neck all the way down through your back, glutes, hamstrings and calves, to the soles of your feet. In cobra you stretch the front of your body, from the front of your neck, chest and shoulders all the way down through your abs, the front of your hips and your quads to the front of your ankles and feet, lengthening the entire back and front of the body. As you switch from downward-facing dog to cobra you strengthen the upper body, core, lower back and glutes. By including this flow into a regular part of your pre-training or match routine you will prepare your body and mind for the demands on the pitch. Focusing on your breath while moving through this flow will enhance your focus and concentration, releasing tension in the body and mind. Integrating these movements regularly into your daily routines will benefit in better posture, improved flexibility and mobility, stronger core and upper body muscles, mental clarity and stress relief.

1. Begin in a tabletop position. Inhale fully and as you exhale lift your hips up high and move into downward-facing dog (see page 48), with your knees slightly bent, spine and arms straight, and palms on the floor. Keep your neck and head relaxed.

2. Take your time here. Pedal your feet, gently moving your heels towards the floor one at a time, for a few deep, slow breaths.

continues overleaf

YOGA FOR FOOTBALLERS

3. On an exhale move into yoga plank (see page 44), holding it for as long as it feels good for you and your body.

4. Keep your body in a straight line, heels above and in line with the base of your toes, and your core muscles activated. Gently shift your weight forward, so your shoulders are above your wrists.

5. When you feel ready, start to slowly lower your body, either halfway or all the way to the floor, keeping your elbows close to your body, untucking your toes, placing the front of your feet on the floor, and straightening your arms as you lift your chest and face upwards (see page 50). Gently press the top of your feet into the floor and you should feel your lower body muscles engaging.

6. You can either do this as one round or, to do a flow of this movement, tuck your toes in, press yourself back up and into a downward-facing dog, and then flow through for a few rounds.

NOTE
Your heels don't necessarily have to lie flat. If the back of your body, particularly your calves, are very tight it might take a while before you can touch the floor with them. If your chest and shoulders are very tight, your hands can be slightly wider apart.

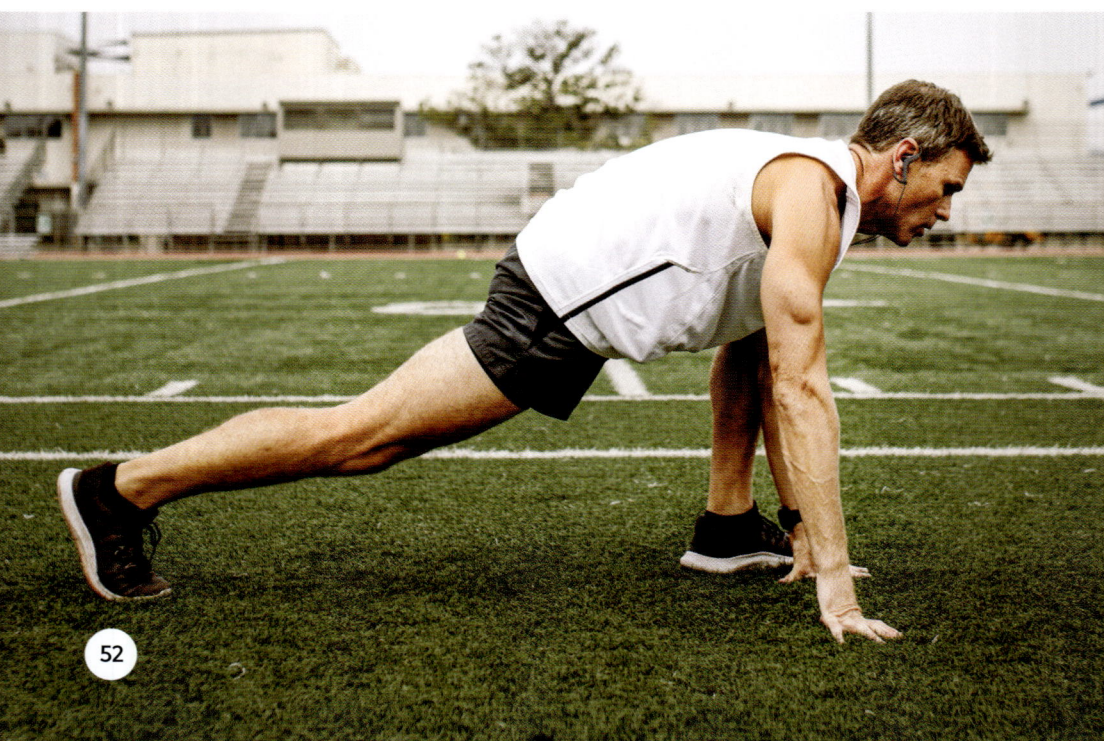

7 WARRIOR 3

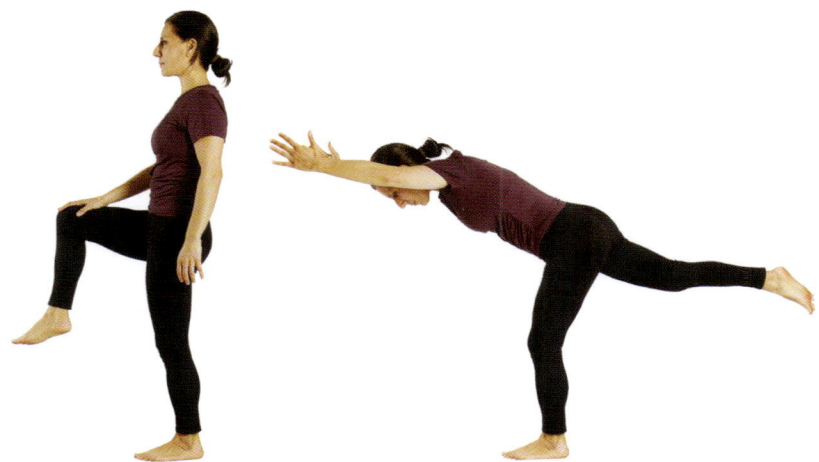

Warrior 3 engages the arms, upper body, lower back, core, glutes and leg muscles. While some of these areas are being strengthened, other areas, like the hamstrings and calves, are also being lengthened. Holding the pose requires concentration and focus, which enhances mental clarity.

This version of warrior 3 is slightly different to the way it is often performed, but I find it much better for players. By bringing the knee up into a 90-degree angle and simultaneously pressing your knee into your hand before extending your leg back, you will involve your core muscles to stabilise your torso and maintain balance, while getting the hip flexor muscles and top of the quads engaged.

If you're new to this pose you may find it easier to start with your arms out to help with balance.

1. Stand upright with your feet hip-width apart and arms at your sides.

2. Inhale and shift all your weight on to your left leg.

3. Exhale, lift your right leg off the ground, bend your knee to 90 degrees and gently press the top of your knee into your right hand for a full breath.

4. Hinge your hips forward, and send your right leg back and behind you, while bringing your upper body forward and parallel to the floor, so you look like a capital letter T from the side.

5. Once in your T, extend your arms forward and in front of you, biceps beside your ears and shoulders relaxed.

6. Think about the front of your hips and make sure your hip bones are both pointing down towards the floor.

7. Keep your gaze on a focus point on the floor and engage your core muscles to maintain stability and balance.

8. Hold the pose for 15 to 30 seconds, while breathing slowly and deeply.

9. To release, slowly bring your right leg back to the floor. Take a moment then repeat on the other side.

8 FOOTBALL STAR

Like the warrior 3, the football star works on balance, strength, stability, and enhancing focus and concentration, which are all very important aspects of preparation for a training session or game.

In this pose we go deeper into the stability of the hips, since one leg is in the air, the outer hip muscles (the abductors) are actively engaged and so are the inner thigh muscles (the adductors). Over time they will strengthen, which leads to better alignment and stability in the hips, and overall lower body strength, which is crucial for reducing the risk of injuries related to imbalance, or instability of the joints, and in preventing certain overuse injuries.

Strengthening the inner thigh muscles – the groins as we call them – is significant in a sport like football where you're frequently called upon to change direction, often very quickly, and the groins play an important role in enabling these smooth and controlled movements.

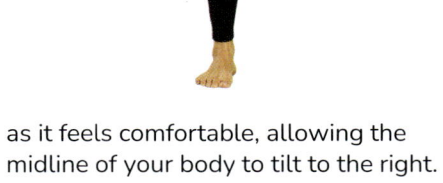

1. Stand upright with your feet hip-width apart and arms relaxed beside your body.

2. Inhale and on the exhale shift all your weight on to your right leg.

3. As you shift your weight on to your right leg, bring both arms up and above your head, palms facing each other, keeping your arms wide apart like a letter V from the front.

4. Start moving your left leg away from the mid-point and to the side, as far as it feels comfortable, allowing the midline of your body to tilt to the right.

5. As you move your left leg away from you, allow your right arm to tilt down, so your body forms a slightly lopsided star shape.

6. Keep your tail bone pointing down and your hip bones pointing forward, so your hips don't rotate. Your shoulder blades should be slightly down and tucked in. Engage your core and gaze forwards. Focus on slow inhales and exhales.

7. Hold this position for 15 seconds or longer if it feels comfortable.

8. To release, slowly bring your left leg back down to the floor and your arms down. Shake your arms and shoulders out and repeat on the other side.

9 HIGH LUNGE FLOW

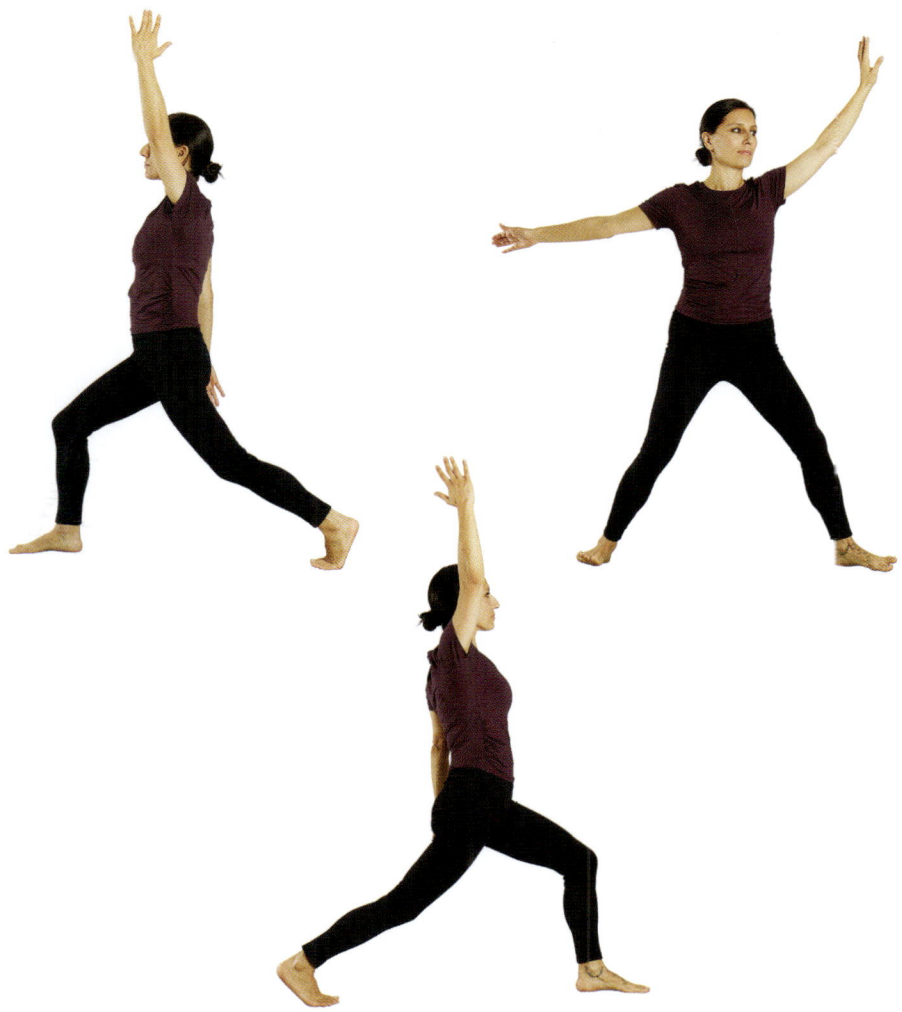

As a footballer, it's always beneficial to gain extra hip mobility before a training session or game. The high lunge flow lengthens the quads and hip flexors, helping to improve the range of motion in the hips, which is crucial for sprinting, changing direction and repetitive kicking.

When performing this dynamic warm-up flow, you also engage and activate your core muscles, improve balance and coordination, and enhance your focus and concentration. These benefits contribute to complete mental and physical preparation, leading to a reduced risk of injury and better overall performance on the pitch.

continues overleaf

YOGA FOR FOOTBALLERS

1. Start in a high lunge position, with your right leg forward and left leg back. Your right knee and right ankle should be in one line, and the middle of your right knee should be in line with your second and third toes on your right foot. Position your right arm beside your body and your left arm overhead and straight up.

2. Inhale and as you exhale transition to the other side of your body, switching your arms mid-sequence, so your left leg is now forward with your left arm beside your body, your right leg back and your right arm is overhead and straight. This is one round.

3. Continue to move through this sequence, transitioning from side to side. You can either stop at each end or flow for a few rounds.

NOTE
Keep an eye on your knee – it should stay in line with your second and third toes, and not move inwards.

OPTIONAL HIGH LUNGE FLOW

Once you have done a few rounds of the high lunge flow, in the starting position you can slowly lower the heel on your back leg to get a bit of lengthening and stretch in the calf muscles and Achilles area.

You could then add a side bend to the overhead arm. This allows you to lengthen the hip flexors a little more, as well as other muscles on the side of your torso, like the lats, and the obliques and intercostal muscles.

This combination of stretches is then even more beneficial, since it not only improves hip mobility, but also enhances flexibility and mobility in the torso, ribcage, shoulders and spine, which all supports movement efficiency.

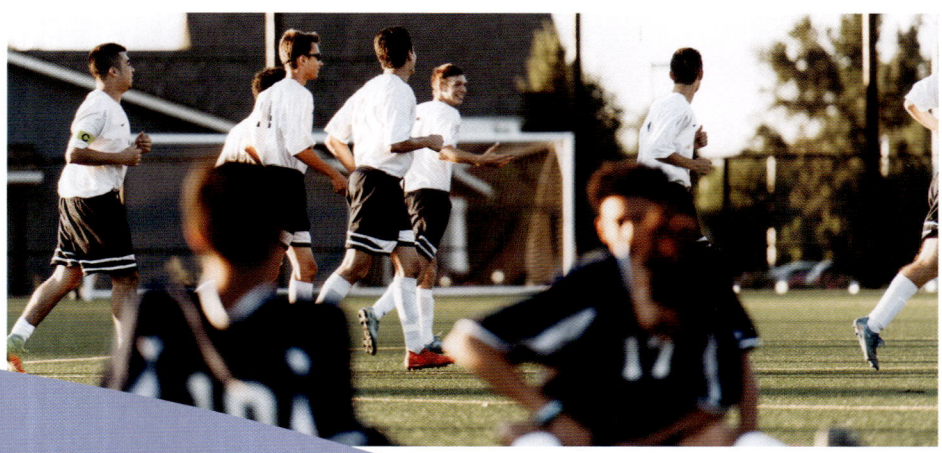

10 FOOTBALL YOGA FLOW

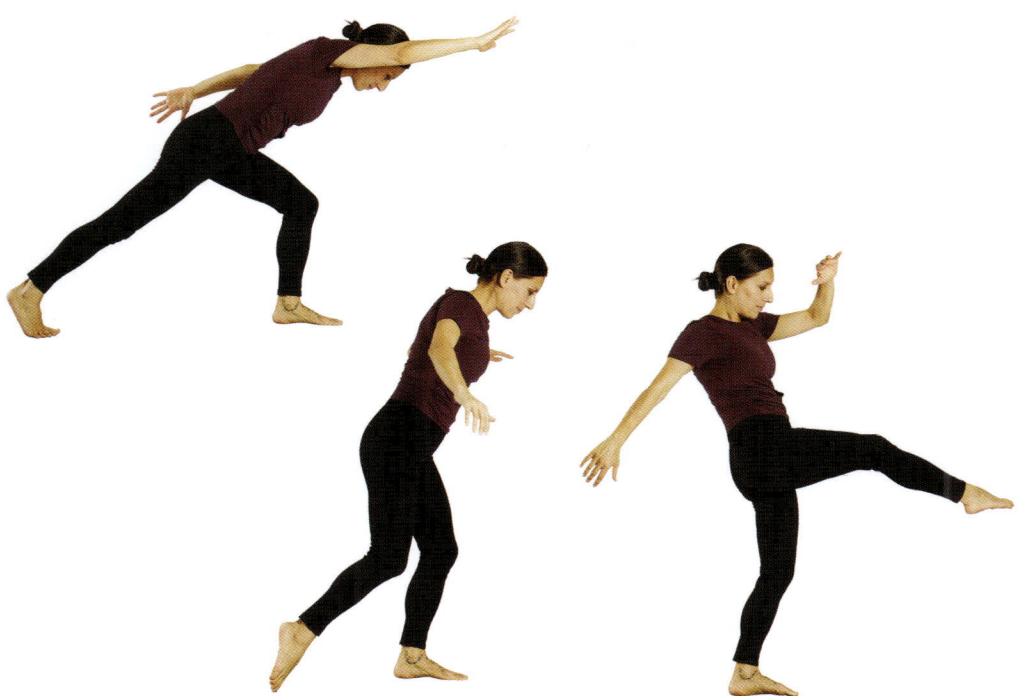

This is a powerful, dynamic movement which can be used in lots of different routines, but it's particularly good as part of a warm-up before a training session or game. It is excellent for increasing strength in the legs and arms, activating the core and glutes, and stabilising muscles, while also improving stability, balance and coordination. It also sharpens focus and concentration.

1. Start in a high lunge position with your right leg back.

2. Lean your upper body forward towards your front leg, so your trunk is parallel to the floor.

3. Extend your right arm forward, so it's also parallel to the floor, bicep beside your ear. Your left arm should also be parallel to the floor and pointing back towards your back foot.

4. Your gaze should be on the floor right below you. Focus on your breath and hold this strong position for a couple of breaths.

5. Now, imagine there is a ball coming at you from in front and in the air, and bring your right leg forward to 'kick' the imaginary ball.

6. Repeat on the other side and do two to three more rounds.

03 POST-TRAINING/ POST-MATCH ROUTINE

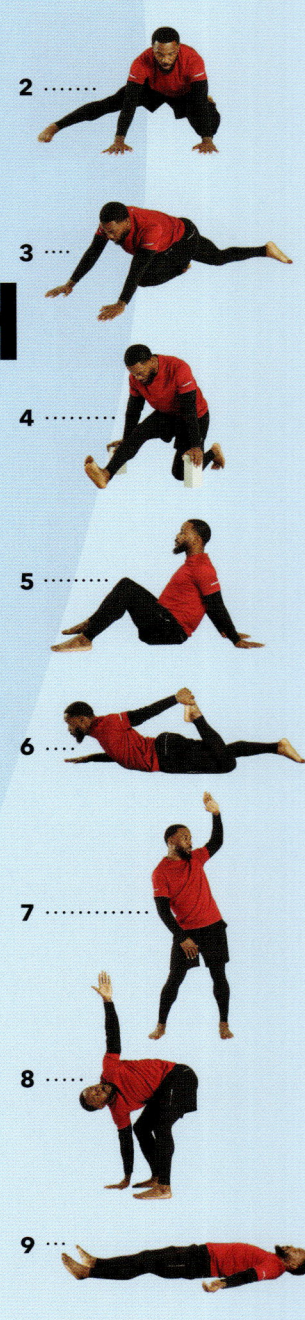

1 Spinal dance .... page 60
2 Modified gate .... page 61
3 Diagonal dynamic pigeon ..... page 63
4 Half split
(toes up and down) .... page 64
5 Letter M movements .... page 66
6 Half frog .... page 67
7 Figure of eight .... page 69
8 Forward bend with twists .... page 70
9 Savasana .... page 72

A good post-exercise recovery routine enhances your overall wellbeing, and feeds into your long-term success and career longevity.

03 POST-TRAINING/POST-MATCH ROUTINE

As you know, after training or a game you can experience a range of physical, mental and emotional feelings. The most common will probably be physical fatigue, which may show up as tightness and tension in your muscles and soft tissue, but if you've really committed yourself you're also likely to be mentally and emotionally exhausted. Recovery is therefore vitally important and you need to start your recovery routine as soon as you can in order to restore your body, mind and emotions, and return them to equilibrium.

So, after a training session or match, your muscles will probably ache and feel stiff. This, of course, is caused by the intensity of your exertion, as well as the accumulation of lactic acid – and the sooner the lactic acid is removed from your system, the sooner these symptoms will disappear and you will start to feel rejuvenated.

In this routine, the poses and movements aid the removal of lactic acid by enhancing your circulation and therefore the delivery of fresh oxygen to your muscles, while stimulating your body's natural detoxification process – its lymphatic drainage system – to effectively flush out toxins and waste products from the system.

Integrating this routine into your training regime will renew your energy and your mental resilience, ensuring you can continue to perform at the same level in the next session or match.

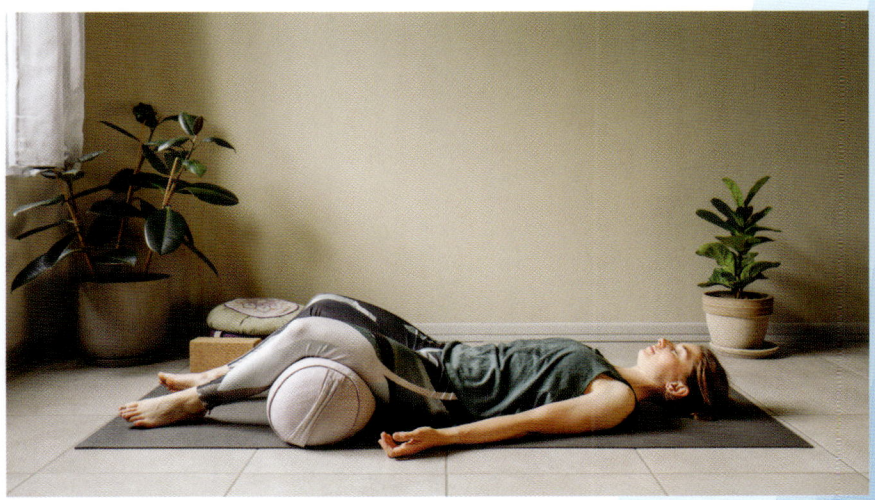

1 SPINAL DANCE

Due to the demands of the sport, most players experience tightness in the lower back and hips from time to time. This simple movement can help improve tension in and around your hips, pelvis, lower back and lower spine, and supports the recovery process by increasing the blood flow to that area. There is no right or wrong way of doing this movement – just flow at your own pace and however that feels good, but while you're moving through this pose imagine your spine dancing.

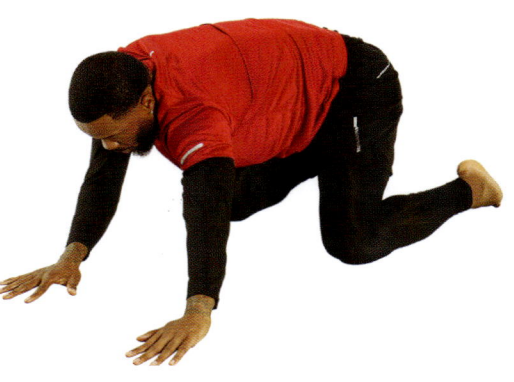

1. Begin on your hands and knees, in a tabletop position. Make sure your wrists, elbows and shoulders are in line, and your knees are below your hips, hip-width apart.

2. Inhale and on the exhale slowly start to move your hips in a circular movement.

3. You can switch between moving clockwise and anticlockwise, and making smaller and bigger circles – whatever feels good and comfortable for you – but create a fluid and smooth movement, with no beginning or end, and focus on your inhales and exhales, breathing deeply and slowly.

4. Move for a few breaths, until you feel your hips and back are starting to loosen up, and your body feels warmer.

5. You can perform this movement for one or a few rounds, shaking your wrists out a little between rounds if you want to.

OPTIONAL SPINAL DANCE

Combining spinal dance with cat and cow (see page 28) can be very effective, so try moving your hips for a few rounds then adding a couple of rounds or more of cat and cow, before going back to your hips, and so on. It is also beneficial to add a few rounds of shoulder circles to release the tension in your upper back and chest muscles, while improving your shoulder mobility.

If you want to build on the previous variations, add a thoracic twist to your spinal dance. This will help improve mobility in your upper and middle back, which is crucial for effective body rotation and also for optimal breathing, since it helps open up the ribcage area and creates more space for the lungs to inflate.

2 MODIFIED GATE

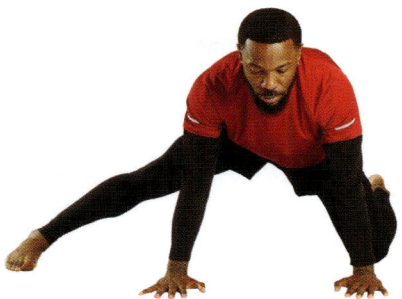 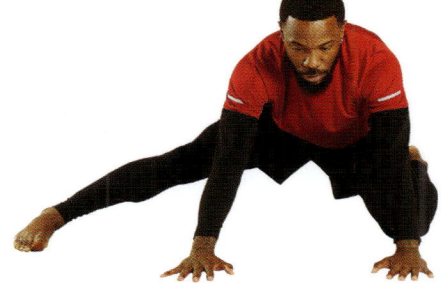

With the spinal dance you have opened up, created good mobility and warmed up your spine, shoulders and hips properly. Now you can go deeper into the range of your hip motion and the flexibility of your groin muscles.

Modified gate is one of my favourite poses and one that I include in all clients' programmes, since it has numerous benefits for footballers and is highly effective for recovery. It effectively lengthens and stretches the adductor or groin muscles, reducing the risk of one of the most common football injuries – groin strain. On the pitch, this can happen due to muscular imbalances, sudden changes of direction and explosive sprint take-offs. Groin strains can greatly impact footballers because they're painful and mean you can't make training.

The lengthening of these inner thigh muscles also improves the overall mobility of the hip joint, leading to a wider range of motion and hence enhancing the mechanics of kicking, and the ability to execute with more power and sharpness when moving on the pitch.

Performing this pose as a part of your post-training or post-match routine helps muscle recovery by releasing the tension in the adductors and surrounding hip muscles, removing lactic acid from those muscles and hence accelerating the recovery process.

1. Begin on your hands and knees, in a tabletop position. Make sure your wrists, elbows and shoulders are in line, and your knees are below your hips, hip-width apart.

2. Extend your right leg to your right side, in line with your hip, with all five toes pointing forward, and the outer edge of your foot and little toe down on the mat and engaged. Your left knee and both palms should be down on the mat. Keep your arms straight, head in line with your spine, and upper body and core lifted and active.

3. Inhale and as you exhale slowly move your body back towards your left heel and back to the starting position.

4. Move backwards and forwards five to six times or longer if your groin still feels tight. Once you have moved a few times and you can feel it loosening up, you can pause and hold the position, focusing on deep and slow breaths.

continues overleaf

5. Once you're done on the right side, slowly bring your leg back into the tabletop position. Repeat on the other side for one or two more rounds.

6. Between sides you can also add the spinal dance (see page 60) for a few breaths or, when you're in the initial position with your leg to the side and in line with your hip, you can add a twist to the pose by opening up towards the same side as the extended leg. Inhale and as you exhale open your chest, twist and extend your arm up towards the ceiling. Pause for a few breaths and slowly return to the middle.

NOTE
It is very common for footballers not to be able to get their little toe all the way down to the floor, so if you can't, don't worry. Think about pressing the outer edge of your foot down as much as possible, just so the inner arch of your foot doesn't collapse, and over time you will eventually be able to get your little toe down.

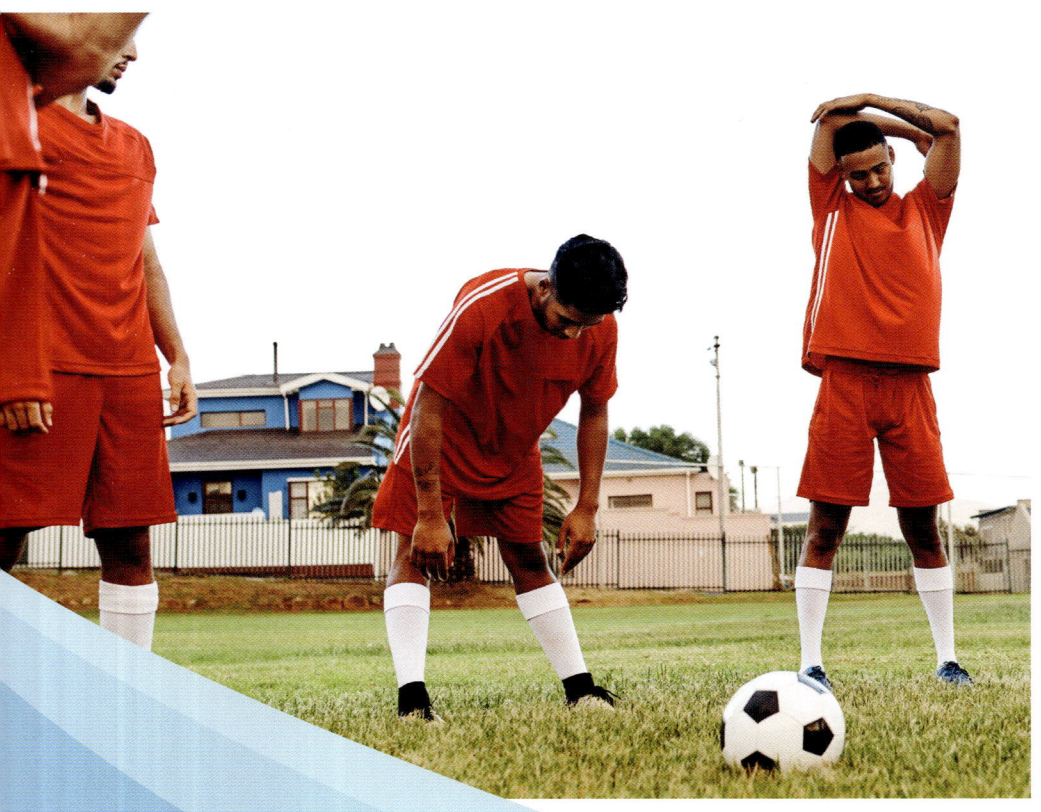

3 DIAGONAL DYNAMIC PIGEON

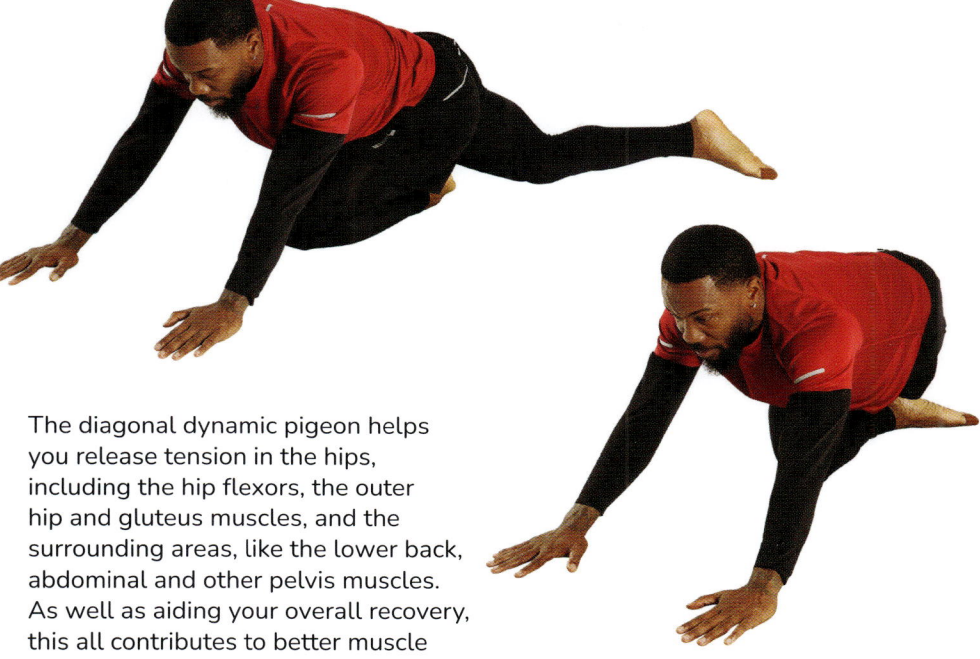

The diagonal dynamic pigeon helps you release tension in the hips, including the hip flexors, the outer hip and gluteus muscles, and the surrounding areas, like the lower back, abdominal and other pelvis muscles. As well as aiding your overall recovery, this all contributes to better muscle elasticity, improved blood flow and greater hip joint mobility, meaning you will move more smoothly on the pitch, and are more likely to avoid hip and groin injuries.

1. Begin on your hands and knees, in a tabletop position. Make sure your wrists, elbows and shoulders are in line, and your knees are below your hips, hip-width apart.

2. Inhale and as you exhale straighten your right leg and move it diagonally back towards your left, as far as it can go and with your back knee down on the floor. Your arms should be straight, your chest and upper body lifted and in line with your head, and your gaze forward.

3. Inhale and come back to the tabletop position.

4. Exhale, and straighten and move your left leg diagonally back and towards your right. That's one round.

5. Do this movement for five to eight rounds, focusing on deep, slow breaths. If possible, allow the length of your breath to be the length of each move.

6. Once you've done these movements for a few rounds, try two to three extra rounds with holds, so once your leg is in the diagonal position, hold the pose for a few deep breaths.

4 HALF SPLIT (TOES UP AND DOWN)

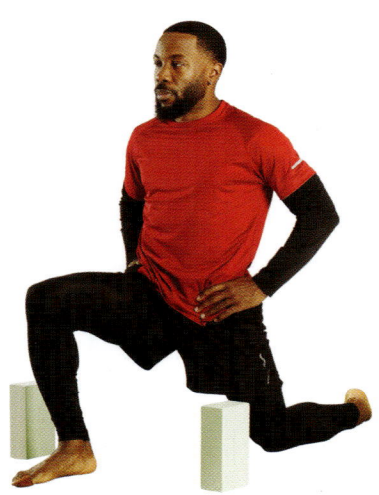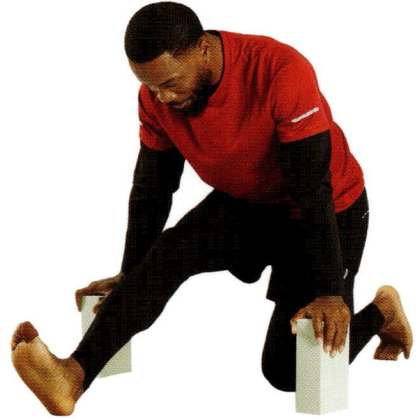

This pose beautifully lengthens the hamstring and calf muscles of the front leg, improving the overall flexibility of these muscles and helping to prevent injuries like strains and tears, which are common in footballers, while also opening up and lengthening the back leg, hip flexors and quad muscles.

It is usually done with the toes of the front leg pointed up and flexed, to support the lengthening on the back of the leg. However, pointing the toes down towards the floor also opens up the front of the ankle and lengthens the front of the shin muscles. These muscles are often tight in footballers, from kicking and running, but they seldom get much attention, so by extending the foot downwards you will really help this area to open up.

1. Start in a low lunge position with your left knee on the mat and right leg forward, your ankle and knee in one line. Keep your hips square.

2. Inhale and as you exhale shift your hips back and straighten your right leg, with your fingers touching the mat, or resting on the blocks, on either side of your front leg.

3. Inhale and flex the toes of your right foot up towards the ceiling. As you exhale, point them down to the floor. The backs of your toes might not touch the mat initially.

4. Once you have moved your toes up and down a few times, keep them pointing upwards, exhale and lean your upper body forward over your right leg. Make sure your spine is nice and long, and your head is in line with your spine.

03 POST-TRAINING/POST-MATCH ROUTINE

5. Stay here for a couple of breaths. If you want to deepen the stretch on the back of the hamstring, flex your foot a little more.

6. Inhale and on the exhale slowly move back to the initial low lunge position, placing your hands on either side of your hips.

7. Engage your core muscles by gently squeezing your belly button towards your spine, keeping your upper body upright, shoulders stacked in line with your hips and your tail bone pointing down towards the floor to maintain a straight line through your spine.

8. Inhale and on your exhale very gently lean your chest and upper body back, without creating too much of a curve in your lower back. Hold this pose for two to three breaths or as long as it feels good.

9. Slowly release and repeat on the other side.

> **NOTE**
> *If you're new to this, and/or very tight at the front of your ankle, it can initially be a bit uncomfortable to point your toes down to the floor.*
>
> You can place blocks or books on either side of you for extra support, or if your hands do not reach the floor. If you have knee issues, you can also fold a blanket and place it under your knee for extra comfort and support.
>
> When in the lunge position, keep your tail bone pointing down towards the floor, so your hips are in neutral, not tilting forwards or backwards, which can sometimes happen. This helps avoid unnecessary strain on the hips and lower back, and also aids engagement of the lower abdominal muscles.

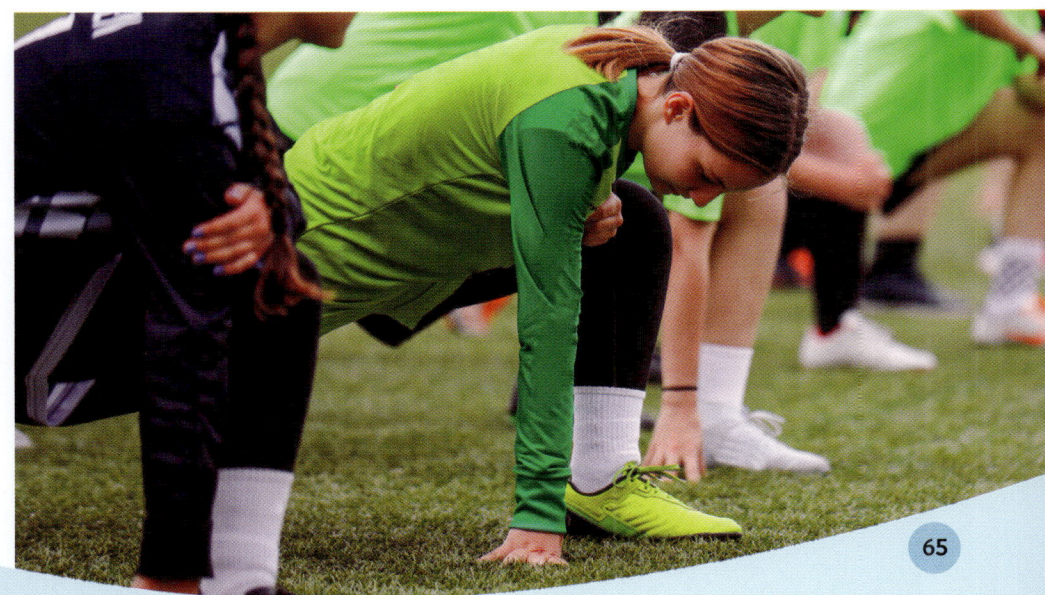

5 LETTER M MOVEMENTS

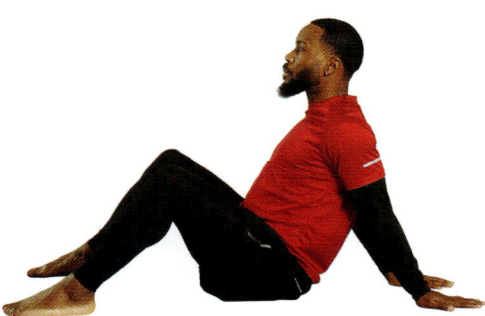
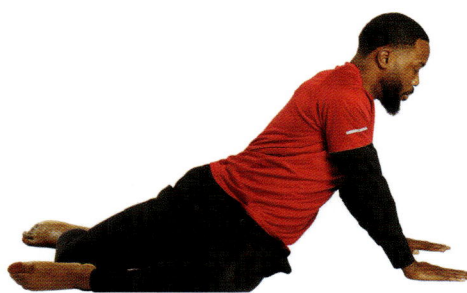

Hips play a very important role in the mechanics of kicking, and having flexible hip joints allows a broader range of motion, which leads to kicks that are more precise and powerful.

You also need a sturdy and flexible spine, which enables smoother, more effective movements on the pitch and reduces stress on the back because it can better absorb the impact from tackles, landing after a header or falls.

This set of movements supports the hips and spine, and helps develop a strong and stable core, and, just like the other poses in this routine, it aids the recovery process by contributing to enhanced circulation and the removal of waste product from the system, thus reducing muscle soreness and fatigue.

1. Sit in the middle of your mat with your knees bent and feet planted on the mat, wider than hip-width apart, and your arms behind you, palms facing down. Keep your spine upright and eyes forwards. From the side, you should look like a capital letter M.

2. Inhale and as you exhale drop both your knees to your left and continue the movement by twisting as far as it feels comfortable to your left, placing your hands behind you on the mat. Look over your left shoulder and behind you if you can. While in your twist your arms should be straight, your upper body and spine nice and long, your head in line with your spine and gaze forward but behind you.

3. Inhale and slowly come back to the middle on an inhale. Then, as you exhale, drop your legs towards your right and twist towards that side too. That is one round.

4. Repeat this movement for another four to five rounds, allowing the length of your breath to be the length of the movement.

5. Then add a few rounds where you pause at the end of the twist, holding the pose for a couple of breaths and going deeper into the twist, while focusing on deep and slow breaths.

6. Once you've done a few rounds with both movement and with a pause, you can lower your upper body all the way to the floor, resting your forehead on the mat, your forearms or making a pillow with your hand.

6 HALF FROG

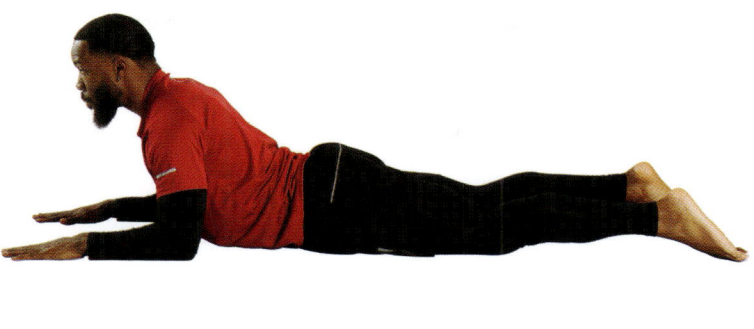

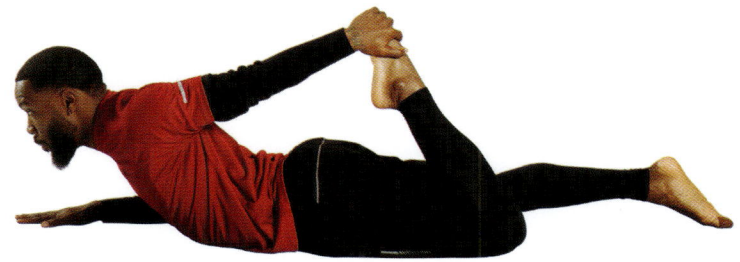

It is now time to target the quadriceps muscles and the front of the body. The half frog supports the flexibility of the quads, providing a deep stretch that helps tension and tightness to release in these muscles and can therefore prevent injuries such as quad strains and tears.

As well as the quads, this pose also lengthens other connective tissue, muscles and fascia of the superficial front line and the deeper anterior line – areas such as the muscles along the front and sides of the neck, the chest, the abs, the deep core, the hip flexors and the front of the ankle. Lengthening these areas is essential for many aspects of the game, including sprinting, changing direction, stride length, more accurate and powerful kicks, and more fluid and effective movement on the pitch.

This pose is therefore an excellent addition to your post-training or post-match routine because it will help your flexibility, reduce the risk of injuries and improve your athletic performance on the pitch, along with enhancing your recovery, maintaining optimal physical condition and extending your longevity as a player.

1. Lie on your front, legs extended and straight behind you, and arms resting beside your body.

2. Inhale and as you exhale gently lift your chest and head away from the floor, placing your forearms on the floor and parallel to each other, shoulders and elbows in one line.

continues overleaf

YOGA FOR FOOTBALLERS

3. On your next exhale bend your left knee, reach your left hand back, take hold of your left foot or ankle and gently bring your heel closer to your buttock until you feel your left quadricep lengthening.

4. Hold this position for four to eight breaths, or longer if it feels good, focusing on deep and slow breaths.

5. Once you're ready to release, do so slowly and come back to the start position. Then repeat on the other side.

NOTE
When in the pose, make sure that the knee and hip on the side you're working on are in line, and the hip doesn't move out to the side. If you can't reach your back foot, you could loop a football sock around your foot to help.

To deepen the 'upper part' of the stretch, you can press into your front forearm and lift your chest and upper abs away from the floor a little, or straighten your arms fully, avoiding lifting your pelvis or hips off the floor and without creating too much compression or discomfort in your lower back.

If the full pose feels too much, you can modify it by not lifting your chest and head away from the floor, but instead resting your forehead on your front forearm or a small pillow.

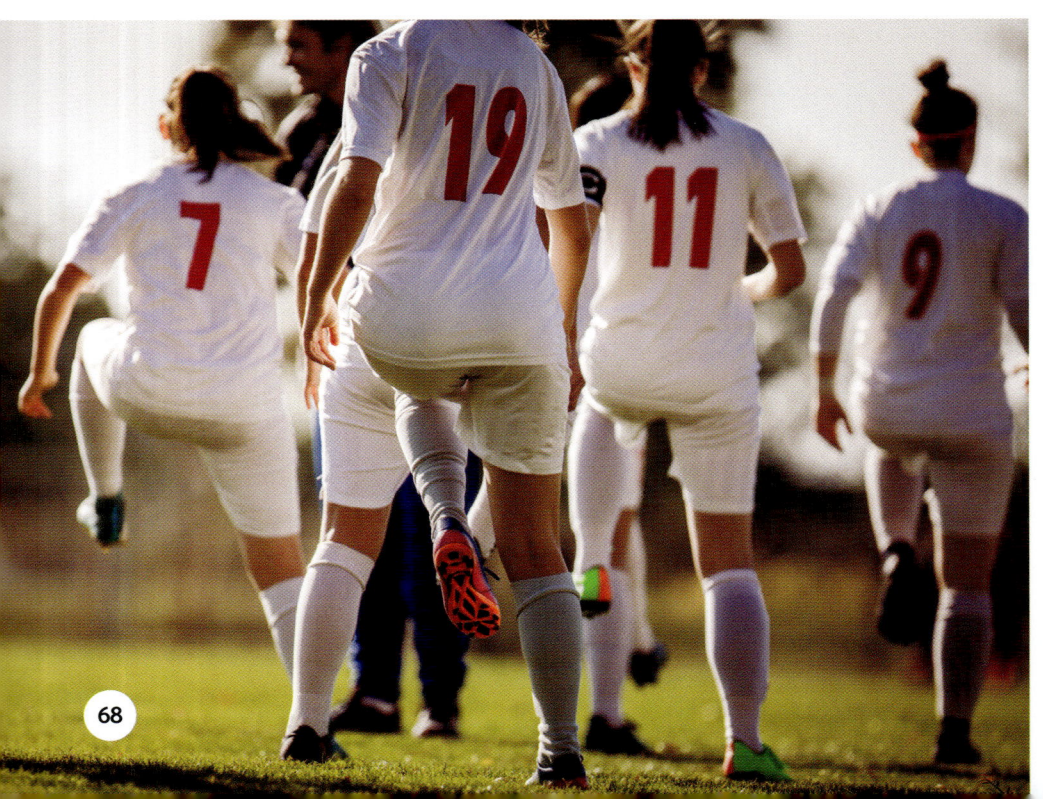

7 FIGURE OF EIGHT

This dynamic flow appears in the morning routine (see page 29), but it is also good as part of a post-training or post-match routine since it stimulates blood flow, which facilitates active recovery and helps remove toxins and metabolic waste. This in turn reduces muscle soreness, improves joint mobility, promotes physical and mental relaxation, enhances nutrient delivery, which is critical for muscle repair and energy restoration, and speeds up the overall recovery process.

1. Stand upright with your feet shoulder-width apart.

2. As you inhale, start moving your hips to the right to begin making a (sideways) figure of eight.

3. As you exhale, shift your weight and your hips to the left.

4. Inhale and move your hips back to the right again.

5. When you find a nice flow, incorporate your arms as well – as you move your hips to the right, move your arms to the right, and so on.

6. Continue for a couple of minutes, until you feel warm and loosened up.

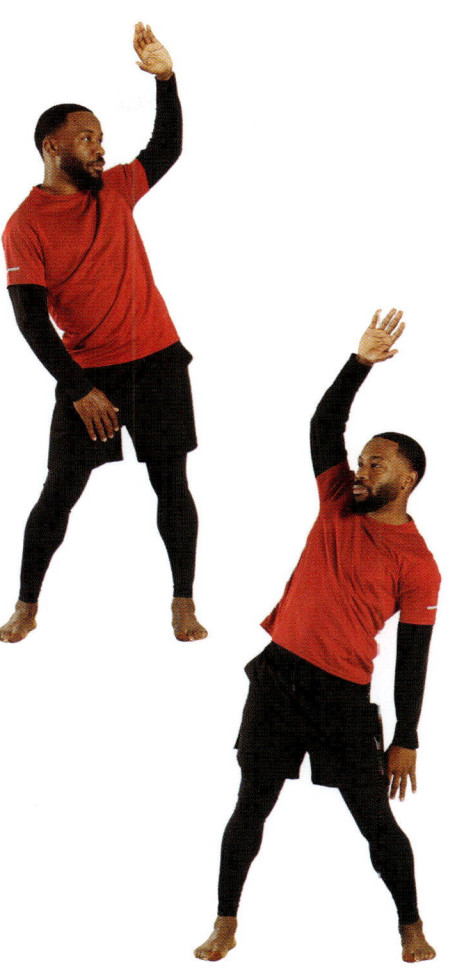

NOTE
You can start these movements with your feet hip-width apart, but as you start loosening up and feeling comfortable, you can move your feet further apart. As you move from side to side, you will also start feeling it in your groin muscles, which makes this a great groin-lengthening exercise too, and therefore this movement is a very good one to incorporate into your pre- or post- training or match routine.

8 FORWARD BEND WITH TWISTS

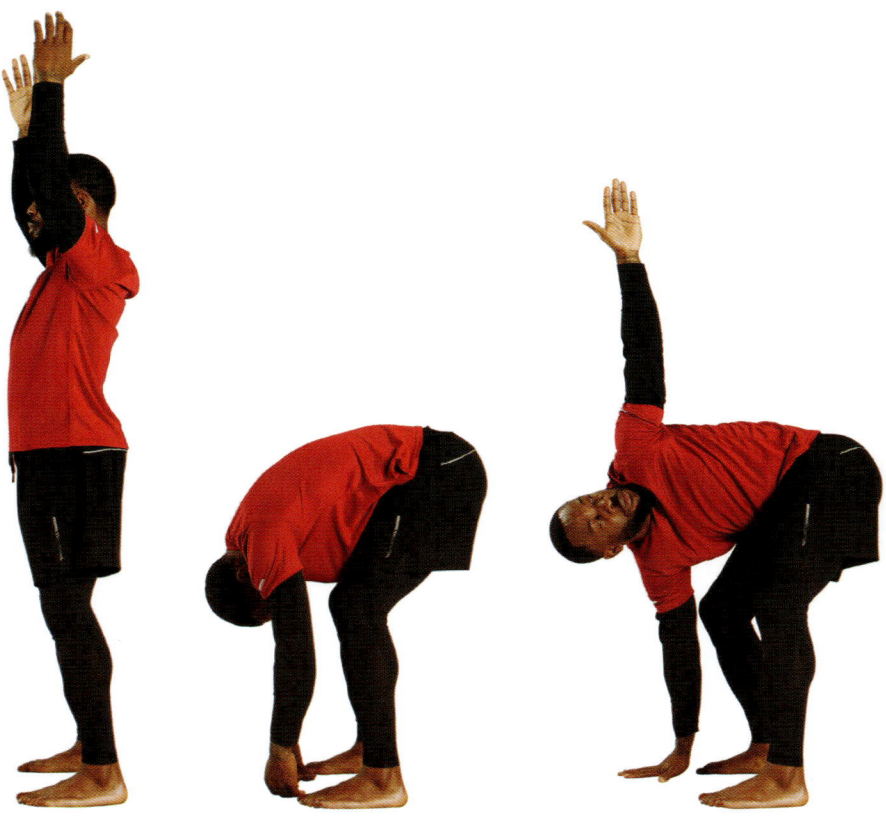

Now your body is properly warmed up, this pose goes a bit deeper into lengthening the hamstrings and releasing tension in the back of the hips, especially the outer hips and lower back area. The added twists contribute to improved spinal flexibility and, as mentioned previously, a flexible spine is crucial to better absorb blows and impacts, and hence lower the risk of back injuries.

However, this pose not only has great physiological benefits, it also has great psychological benefits. In the forward bend your head is below your heart and your parasympathetic nervous system is activated, which stimulates relaxation and thus recovery. Your stress hormones are lowered, helping to create a feeling of calm in the body and mind, yet at the same time, because of this enhanced blood flow to the brain, you can feel alert, energised and more awake. This is particularly valuable after an intense training session or a game.

03 POST-TRAINING/POST-MATCH ROUTINE

1. Start with your legs hip-width apart.

2. Inhale and bring your arms out to the side and up above your head.

3. Exhale and fold forward, keeping your knees slightly bent, so your fingers can reach the floor.

4. Stay in your forward bend for a breath or two.

5. Inhale and on the exhale bend your right knee. With your right fingers or hand on the floor, inhale and on the exhale twist and open your left chest, arm and side of your face towards the left. Straighten your left leg and keep your hips square.

6. Hold the twist for the full exhale or another breath, before slowly coming back to the middle and allowing your head to relax and be heavy again.

7. Repeat the twist on the other side.

8. This pose can be just a movement, you can pause at each end or you can mix movements and pause, for five to eight repetitions or as many as feels good.

NOTE
When performing the twist, if you feel a lot of tension in your legs or are very new to this movement, you can bend both knees slightly. Otherwise, I suggest keeping one knee bent and the other one (on the side you're twisting towards) straight. This will deepen the twist and allow more lengthening in the hamstrings and outer hip muscles on that side.

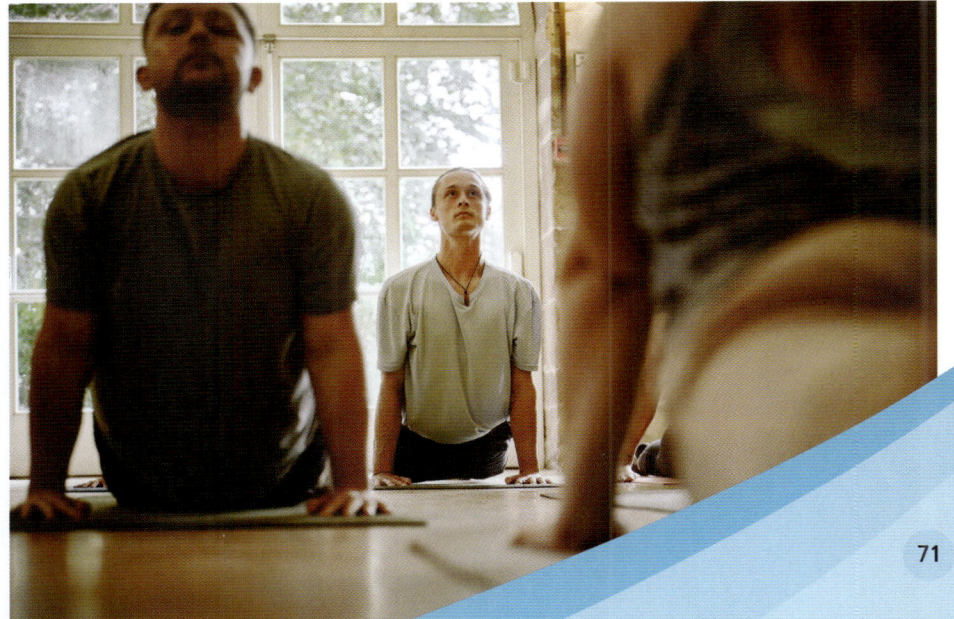

9 SAVASANA

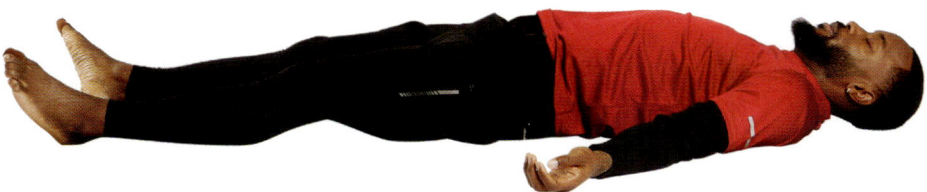

Due to its benefits for mental and physical recovery and relaxation, and nervous system regulation and balance, with the savasana (also called the corpse pose), you can finally transition from intensity to a state of total rest and healing. It allows the heart to slow down, supporting cardiovascular recovery. It also relaxes all muscle groups and encourages full-body relaxation, preparing the body for a restful state and thus better sleep quality.

You can add savasana as the final relaxation part of any routine, since it truly allows a sense of accomplishment, leaving you feeling peaceful and rejuvenated at the same time, knowing that you have given your all and therefore will recover efficiently and feel at your best for the next training session or game.

1. Lie on your back, arms beside but slightly away from your body, palms facing up and legs hip-width apart.

2. Bring your hands to the back of your head, gently lift your head up and lengthen the back of your head as if you're straightening the skin on the back of your neck. This is almost like giving yourself a double chin.

3. Close your eyes and start focusing on your inhales and exhales, and the movement of your breath. Allow your body and mind to relax. Notice how you feel now compared to when you started this routine.

4. Start by staying in savasana for five minutes and then over time progress to longer.

5. When you feel ready to come out of the pose, deepen your breathing and slowly move your fingers and toes to awaken your body. Gently bring your knees up, hugging them in towards your chest and moving from side to side, before rolling on to one side for a few breaths. Then very slowly press yourself up into a seated position and then stand up. Do not stand up or get out of savasana too quickly, but take your time to adjust to being upright.

MODIFIED SAVASANA

Practising savasana with a bolster under your knees is an excellent way to enhance comfort and deepen relaxation. The bolster supports the legs, relieving pressure on the lower back and allowing the body to fully release tension. You can stay in this pose for longer to maximise the restorative benefits. This pose can also be a soothing addition to your evening routine, helping you unwind and prepare for restful sleep.

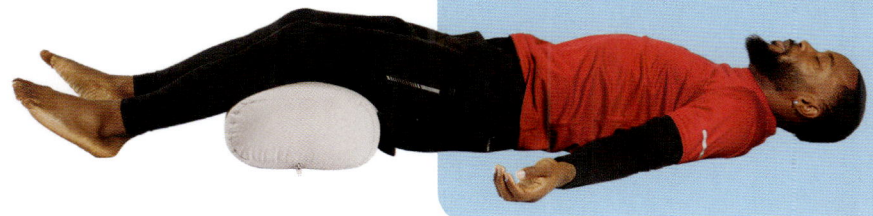

04 EVENING ROUTINE

1. Thoracic book opening .... page 76
2. Supine twist .... page 77
3. Reclined butterfly .... page 78
4. Pigeon .... page 79
5. Child's pose .... page 80
6. Legs up the wall .... page 81
7. 4-7-8 breathing .... page 83

An evening routine that includes calming poses and breathwork can be one of the best practices for the overall wellbeing and long-term health of any footballer.

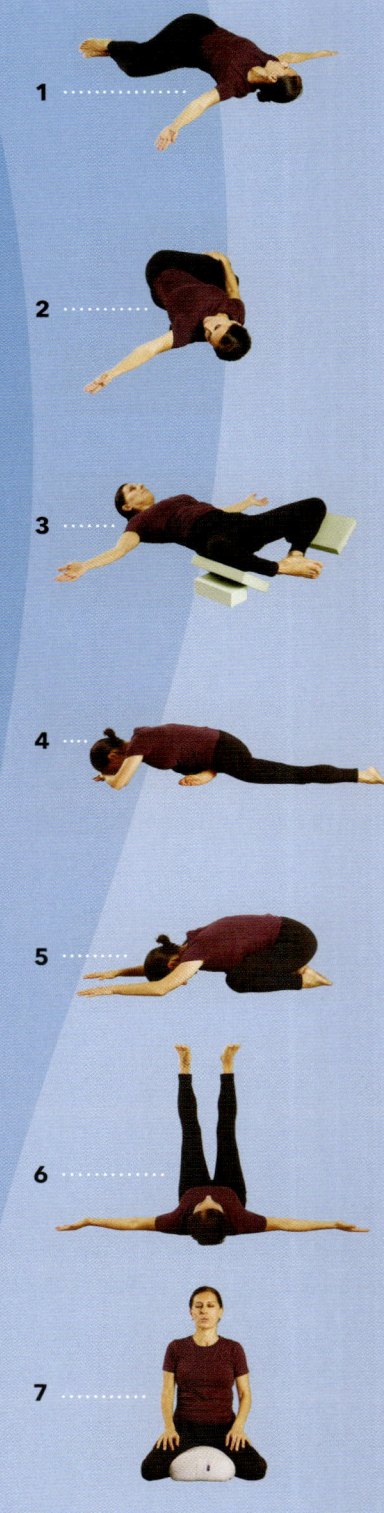

The poses and breathwork in this routine share a common calming effect while enhancing your overall flexibility by gently stretching out and creating space in the areas of your body most impacted by football. All these exercises assist in muscle relaxation, too, which is essential after long days of intense training sessions, games and travel.

This routine also focuses on promoting spinal mobility and alignment, which is critical for footballers. Improved spinal mobility allows the body to move smoothly and efficiently, enhancing performance. Additionally, this routine optimises recovery by releasing tension and increasing blood flow in the spinal area.

There is a focus on slow, deep breathing, leading to enhanced restorative and calming effects, and it also helps improve your breathing by allowing your ribcage to fully expand, giving your lungs more space to function at their full capacity. This not only supports stamina, but is crucial for long-term health, too.

In addition, this routine can play a crucial role in improving sleep quality by preparing your body and mind for rest. The calming effects of these poses, combined with deep breathing, can reduce anxiety and mental fatigue, ensuring you wake up refreshed and focused.

Like all aspects of training, the benefits of this routine are progressive. Regular practice can lead to improved flexibility, reduced injury risk and enhanced mental clarity over time. Incorporating this routine into your daily life will help maintain a balanced state of body and mind, giving those who engage in it regularly a significant advantage.

1 THORACIC BOOK OPENING

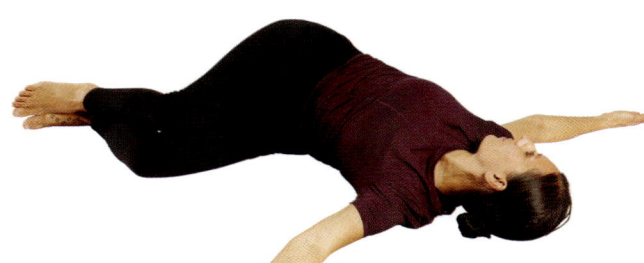

The thoracic spine consists of larger and stronger vertebrae than the cervical (neck) and lumbar (lower back) spine. It contributes to overall stability of the thoracic spine and provides essential support for the ribcage (which is attached to the thoracic vertebrae). It also helps protect important organs such as the lungs and the heart.

By nature and because of its anatomical function, there is limited movement and mobility in this area of the spine, so it is therefore very important to integrate mobility exercises like the thoracic book opening into daily routines.

Due to the nature of football, where a lot of running, changes of direction and twisting leads directly to overuse and tightness in the thorax and the surrounding soft tissue, it is therefore crucial for players to stretch and release tension in this area at the end of the day.

1. Lie on your left side with your legs bent and on top of each other, knees in line with your hips, arms on top of each other and extended straight in front of you.

2. Inhale and on your exhale raise your right arm up and move it in the air over to your right side, as if you're drawing a semi-circle from left to right. Allow your arm to reach all the way to the floor, or as far as it goes, on your right side.

3. Allow your head and spine to rotate with the movement and look towards your right hand.

4. Pause here in your 'open book' position for a breath or two and notice where there is tension.

5. On the next exhale, bring your right arm back to the left one.

6. Repeat this movement eight to twelve times or for as long as it feels good. Then repeat on the other side.

NOTE
As you move through this movement, think about moving the whole of your torso, rather than only your arm, so when you're in 'open book' position, your chest is facing the ceiling.

If your top knee lifts away from the bottom one, gently keep it down with one hand or allow it to lift if that feels better. Find what is most comfortable for you.

It can also be nice to do a few faster repetitions and a few that you pause and hold in 'open book' position.

2 SUPINE TWIST

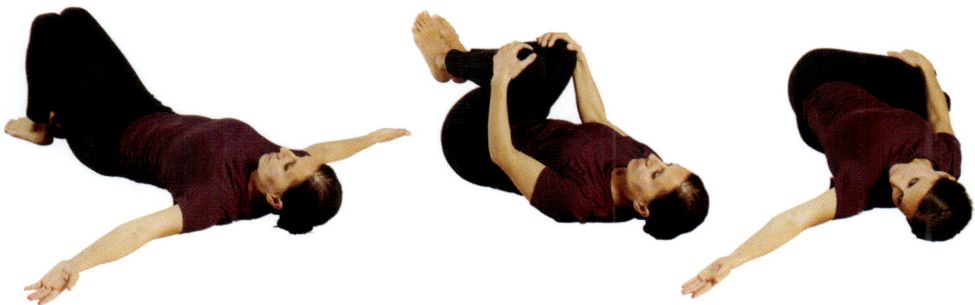

Though the positioning of the supine twist might look similar to that of the thoracic book opening, the two do serve slightly different purposes, even though both support and help maintain a healthy and flexible spine.

This pose will help you wind down and is great to incorporate into your evening routine. It gently opens up, stretches and releases tension in the hips, spine and lower back, while also elongating the shoulders and chest, thus creating more space in the lung area and allowing the breath to move more freely, which promotes calmness and relaxation for body and mind.

NOTE
If you have long-term lower back issues, when performing this pose it will be gentler on your lower back if, instead of hugging your knees into your chest, you allow your feet to stay on the floor, with your legs bent at the knees. Then, when you move them to the side, there won't be any potential jerking in your lower back area. Complete the rest of the steps as described.

1. Lie on your back with your knees bent, feet on the floor. Open your arms out to your sides, creating the shape of a capital letter T.

2. Bend your knees up towards your chest and gently hug them in, but keep your upper body and head on the floor.

3. Inhale and as you exhale gently lower your legs to your right, resting your left arm back on the floor, right hand on top of your left leg, and without lifting your upper body.

4. Inhale and as you exhale look towards your left hand.

5. Hold this position for five to ten breaths, or longer if that feels good, focusing on deep and slow breaths.

6. To release, on an exhale slowly come back to the middle. Repeat on the other side.

3 RECLINED BUTTERFLY

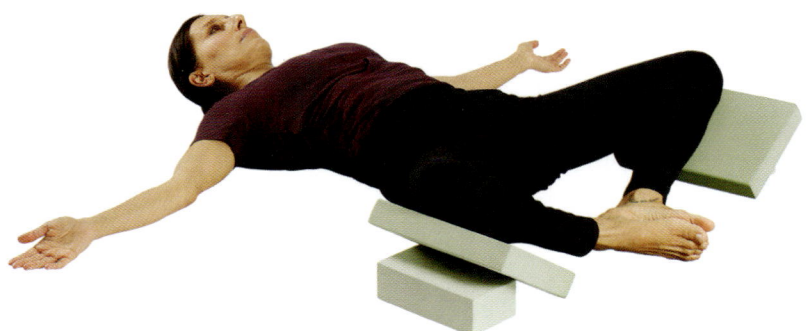

Football is a sport that involves a great number of lateral movements, such as changes of direction, cutting and shuffling but also kicking, acceleration and deceleration. The groin area is heavily engaged in all these movement patterns, so high demands are placed on the adductor muscles, and groin injuries, especially strains, are among the most common for footballers.

The reclined butterfly is a gentle hip opener, which will release tension in the groin and hips, promote blood flow and circulation to this area, and help the muscles to relax and recover. The pose also has a calming and restorative effect on the nervous system, and hence is great to perform in the evening to promote better and more restful sleep.

1. Place blocks or pillows on either short side of your mat, in line with your knees.

2. Lie on your back with your legs straight.

3. Inhale and as you exhale bend your knees, keeping your feet flat on the mat.

4. On the next exhale, allow your knees to fall open and drop out towards the blocks. Allow the soles of your feet to touch.

5. Keep your arms at your side, palms facing up, and your eyes closed if that feels comfortable. Focus on deep and slow breaths.

6. Hold the pose for five to ten breaths, or longer if it feels good, allowing your body to relax into the pose with each exhale.

NOTE
Make sure you have enough blocks or pillows under your knees to support your groin, so you can relax into the pose rather than feeling an intense stretch. Equally, you don't want your knees to be too high up, since that way the groin and hip area won't open up properly. Find a balance that works for you, remembering that it's common for one side of your groin to be tighter than the other.

4 PIGEON

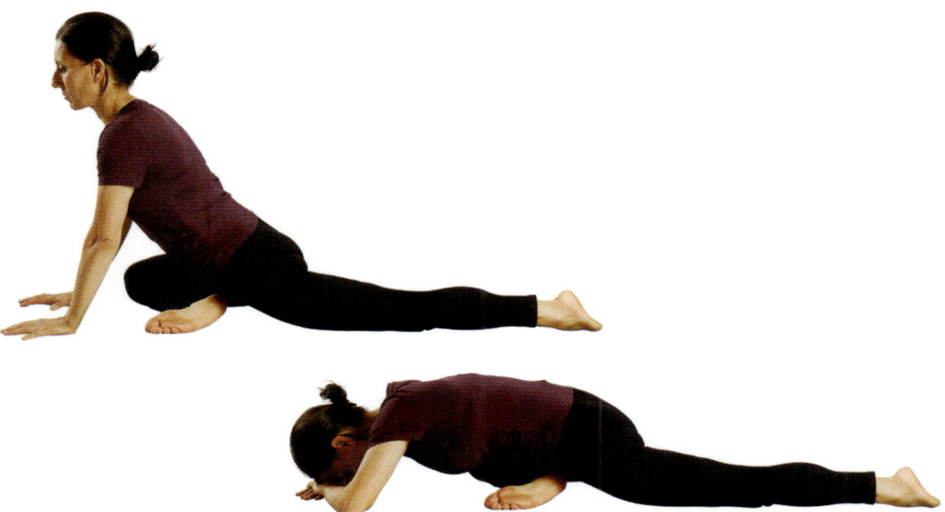

This pose is another great one for healthy hips. It helps to lengthen and release tension in the hip flexors, the outer hip and gluteus muscles, and the lower back, which all contribute to more space and mobility in the hip area. This aids smooth movement on the pitch and helps prevent injuries, but also eases discomfort and contributes to overall relaxation.

The pigeon is versatile and can be used as part of many different routines, but it is included here because it is a powerful pose and, when performed with mindful breathing, it can be used as a tool to calm the body and mind, and bridge you from an active to a peaceful state, ready for a restful night's sleep.

1. Begin on your hands and knees, in a tabletop position. Make sure your wrists, elbows and shoulders are in line, and your knees are below your hips, hip-width apart.

2. Inhale and on your exhale slide your right knee forward towards your right hand. Angle the lower part of your right leg so your foot is near your left hand.

3. Straighten and slide your left leg back, making sure the front of your hips are in line and square.

4. Lower your upper body to the floor, leaning over your right leg. Find a position that is comfortable for you. Either rest your forearms on the mat and lift your chest away from the floor or allow your arms and body to gently fall all the way down. You can make a pillow with your hands or rest your forehead on the floor.

5. Hold the pose for five to twenty breaths, focusing on deep and slow breaths. Repeat on the other side.

5 CHILD'S POSE

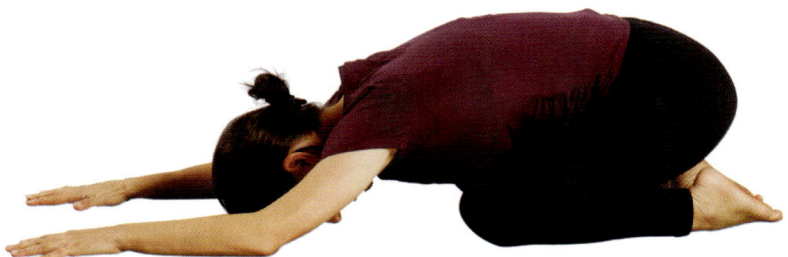

The child's pose is a wonderful restorative pose that can be performed at any time of the day, especially when you feel you need a moment to calm the mind and release stress. This pose not only encourages relaxation, but also stretches and releases any residual tension in the lower back, hips and surrounding areas, so it is ideal for unwinding and prepares you for a good night's sleep.

1. Come on to your mat on your hands and knees. Move your knees apart slightly wider than your hips, your big toes touching behind you (you shouldn't feel any pain in your knees when performing this pose).

2. Inhale and as you exhale move your hips back towards your heels, allowing your belly to rest in between your thighs. Place your forehead on the floor.

3. Keep your arms extended in front of you on the mat or beside your body if that feels better.

4. Close your eyes. Relax your shoulders and jaw. Focus on deep and slow breaths, allowing your body to sink deeper into the pose with each exhale.

5. Hold this pose for five to twenty breaths, or longer if it feels good.

MODIFIED CHILD'S POSE

An excellent restorative variation is to use a bolster under your chest and belly for support. This provides deeper relaxation and encourages a sense of calm. Stay in this pose for three to five minutes, focusing on slow, deep breaths to enhance the calming effects.

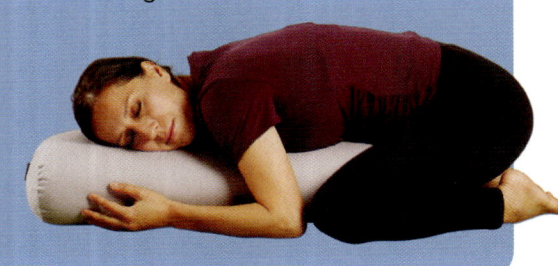

6 LEGS UP THE WALL

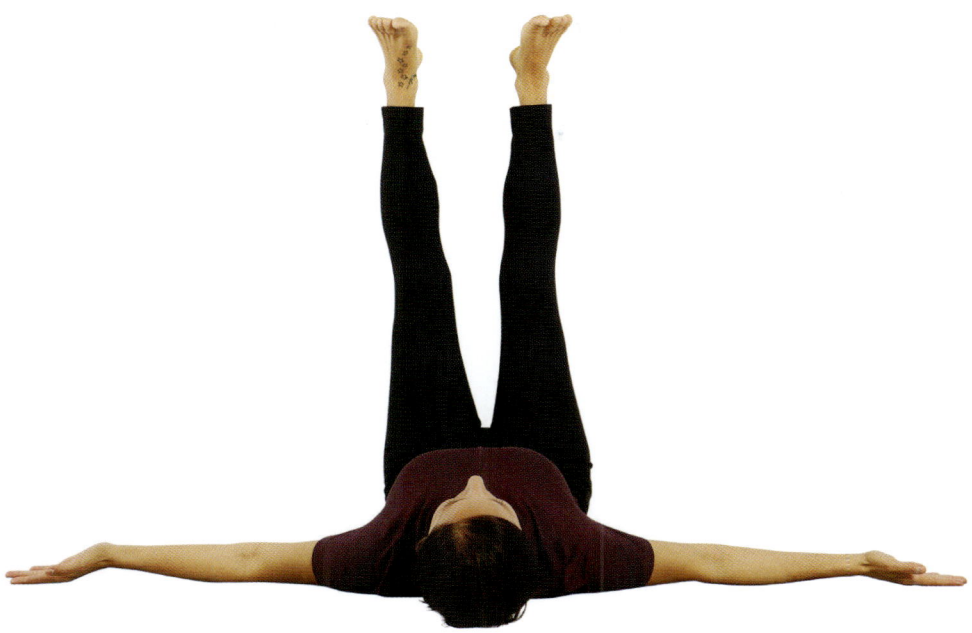

Legs up the wall is another great restorative 'evening' pose that is excellent to perform in the last hour before going to bed. It is a highly beneficial pose that supports multiple body systems and encourages overall health and wellbeing.

By elevating your legs above your heart, you will help your cardiovascular system to return blood flow back to the heart, without the heart having to do it itself, as it does if you're, for example, standing up or sitting down.

With your legs raised and inverted, and with the assistance of gravity, this pose also helps to stimulate the lymphatic system to enhance the process of clearing toxins and waste products, like lactic acid, out of the system. An accumulation of lactic acid can lead to muscle soreness and fatigue, so this pose is excellent for recovery purposes.

It also activates the parasympathetic nervous system, which is responsible for your body's rest and digest functions. This in turn helps you to relax and feel calm in your body and mind, and it enhances the functions of your digestive organs, so your body digests food more efficiently.

1. Sit on the floor near a wall, facing it, with your hips close to the wall and your legs extended.

2. Inhale and on your exhale swing your legs up the wall, lowering your head, the back of your shoulders and your back to the floor.

continues overleaf

3. Ideally your buttocks should be as close to the wall as possible. If this doesn't feel comfortable, or you find it difficult to keep your legs straight, you can shuffle away from the wall.

4. Once you find a comfortable position, place your arms beside your body, palms facing up and eyes closed. Focus on deep and slow breaths.

5. Hold the pose for five to ten minutes (if you're new to the pose, five minutes is fine to start with) or longer once you're used to practising it regularly.

6. When you're ready to release, slowly lower your legs down to one side and stay on your side for a few breaths before getting up.

NOTE
For extra comfort you can put a blanket or a bolster under your hips. This will ease the lower part of your spine and lift your hips a little, which can help with the pose.

It is not uncommon to experience pins and needles or tingly sensations in your legs while in this pose. This can be because of how you have positioned your legs and a nerve or a blood vessel could be being compressed. If this happens it could mean that you have spent long enough in the pose – in which case come out of it. Alternatively, you may need to adjust your position by, for example, moving away from the wall or turning your legs into butterfly legs by bringing the soles of your feet together and letting your knees fall open to the sides (as in the reclined butterfly – see page 78), which will work to lengthen your groin muscles as well.

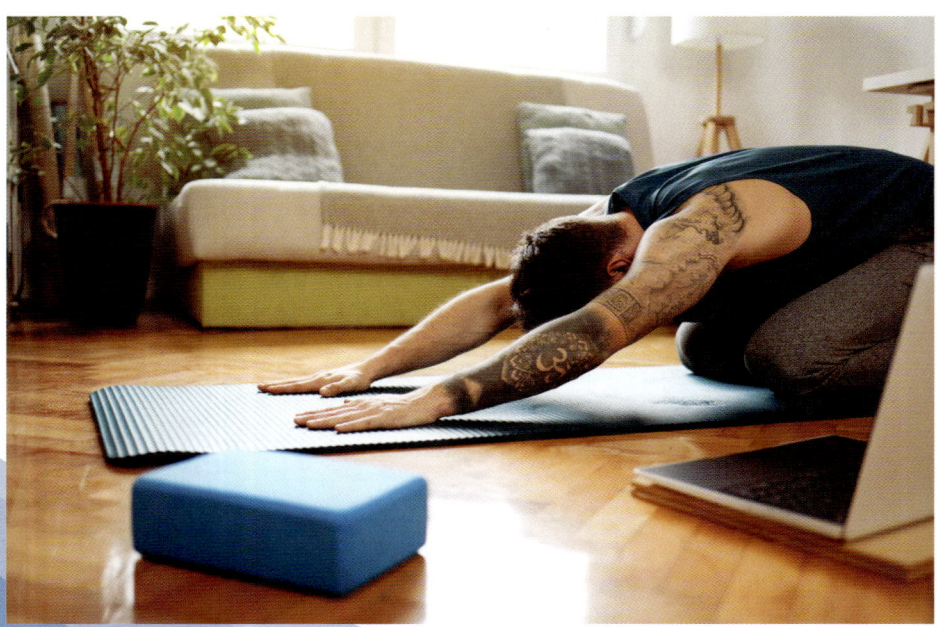

7 4-7-8 BREATHING

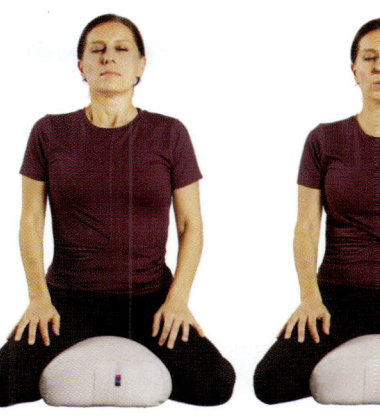

The 4-7-8 breathing technique is a powerful relaxation tool and one that all footballers can really benefit from. The lengthened phase of the exhale stimulates the parasympathetic nervous system, which helps lower the stress in the body and mind, promotes relaxation and therefore helps you fall asleep faster.

Since this breathwork is a profound rhythmic breathing technique and has the extended exhalation part, which helps expel more carbon dioxide, it also enhances the efficiency of oxygen exchange by promoting deeper and more efficient breathing patterns, contributing to improved endurance and stamina, quicker recovery and overall enhanced athletic performance.

Oxygen exchange is the process in which oxygen moves from the air we breathe into our bloodstream, while carbon dioxide moves out of our bloodstream into the air we exhale. It is a process that primarily takes place in the lungs and it is a very important one for good health and overall wellbeing.

1. Sit in a chair or sit or lie on your mat or a bolster. If you're in a seated position make sure your spine and back are straight, chin parallel to the floor, eyes closed, mouth slightly open, and face and shoulders relaxed.

2. Take a couple of full breaths, breathing in and out, allowing yourself to 'arrive' in the here and now.

3. Breathe in slowly and quietly through your nose, with your mouth closed, for a count of four.

4. Hold your breath for a count of seven.

5. Slowly exhale out through your mouth for a count of eight.

6. This completes one round. Repeat this cycle for four to six rounds.

NOTE
If you're new to breathwork it is advisable to start slowly and to listen to your body. You may modify the counts and start with a simpler technique, for example 4-5-6, and then gradually progress.

AVOID IF...
You have respiratory conditions; cardiovascular issues; severe anxiety; other medical conditions such as epilepsy or vertigo; or you're pregnant. If you have any of these conditions or any health concerns, speak to your doctor or health care provider before doing 4-7-8 breathing or any of the breath techniques in this book.

PART TWO

TARGETED ROUTINES

05 Hip routine .... page 86
06 Hamstring routine .... page 102
07 Lower back routine .... page 118
08 Core routine .... page 132
09 Relaxation routine .... page 146

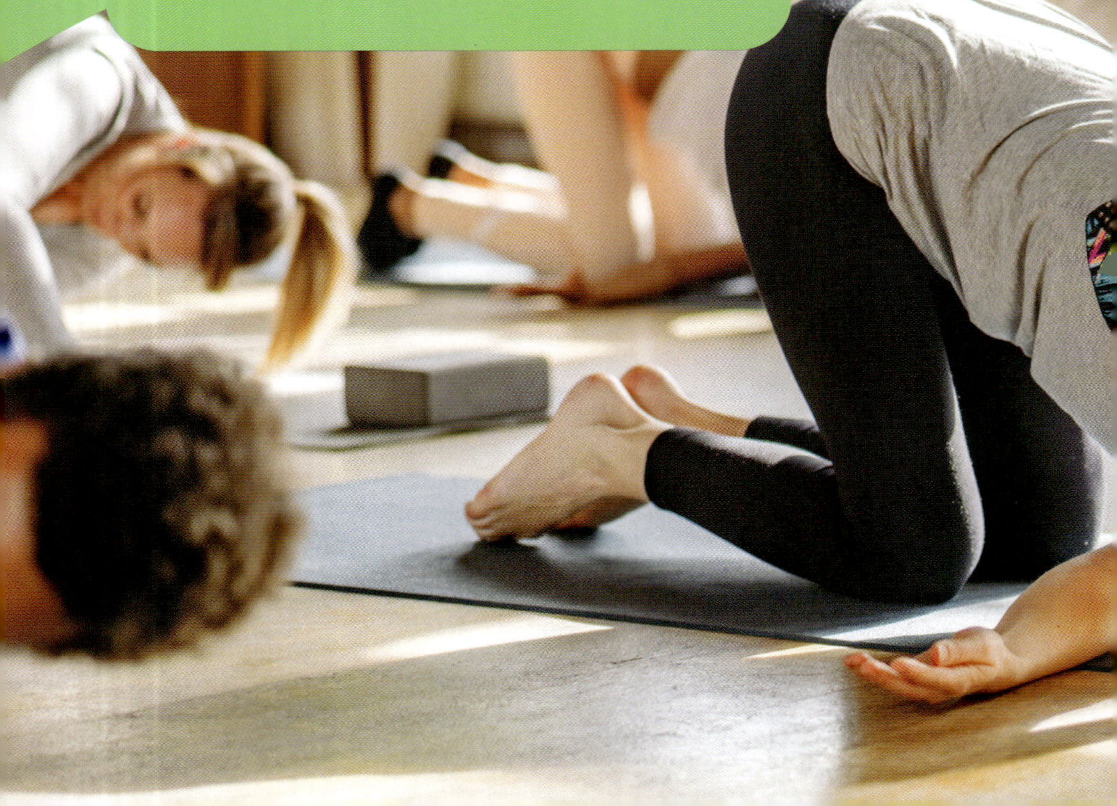

These five routines are designed to target specific areas of your body and can be incorporated into your practice as needed, depending on your individual focus areas, and your unique needs and circumstances. They are versatile and can be practised as a continuous flow, where the postures seamlessly transition from one to the next, or you can select individual poses and integrate them into your daily routines or swap them with exercises from the essential routines in Part One.

I recommend you explore these routines and experiment with what works best for you at different times. For instance, if you're recovering from an injury or have limitations that prevent you from performing the full daily routines, exercises from these targeted routines can be particularly beneficial. They offer targeted support when you need to address tightness in specific areas, focus on rehabilitation or prioritise relaxation.

Integrating these targeted routines into your practice will help you achieve a balanced yoga programme that addresses the needs of both your body and mind, whether in response to the challenges of football or everyday life.

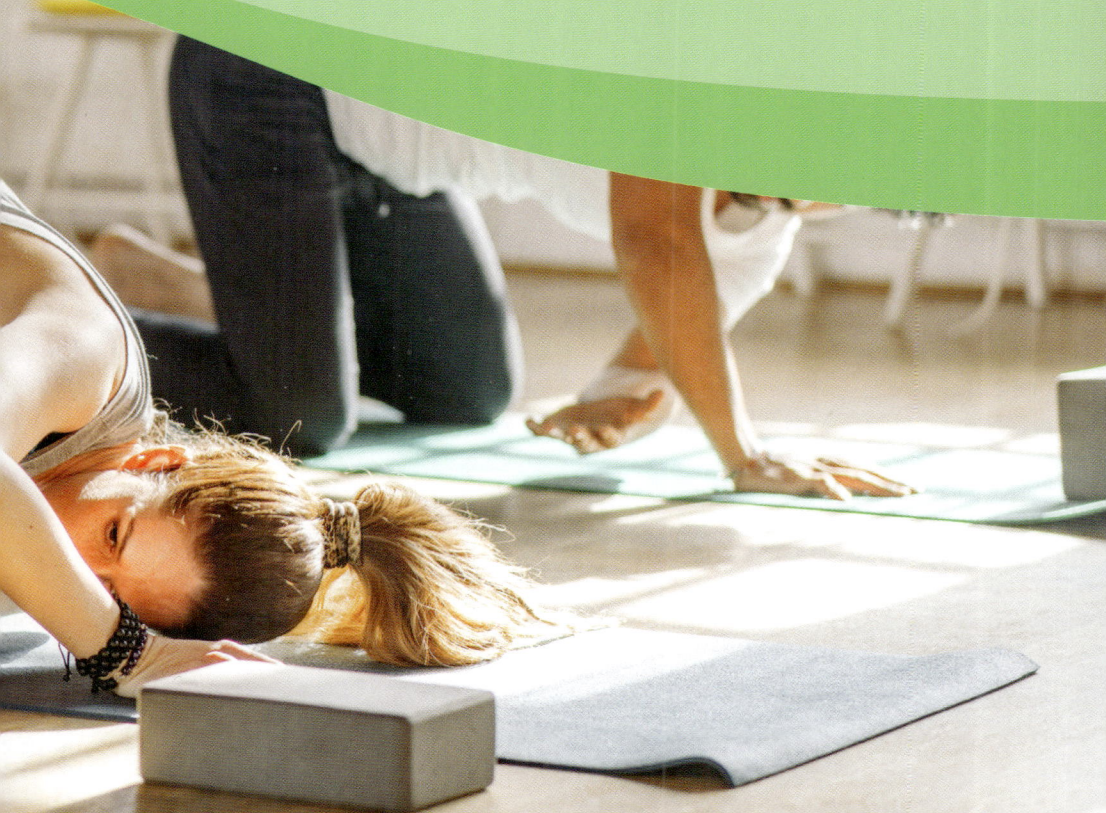

05 HIP ROUTINE

1. Cat and cow .... page 88
2. 90/90 with movement ...... page 89
3. Pigeon with twists .... page 90
4. Lizard .... page 92
5. Frog .... page 94
6. Warrior 1 .... page 96
7. Tree .... page 98
8. Half lord of the fish .... page 100

Football is a physically very demanding game, which means acute and chronic hip injuries are very common among players.

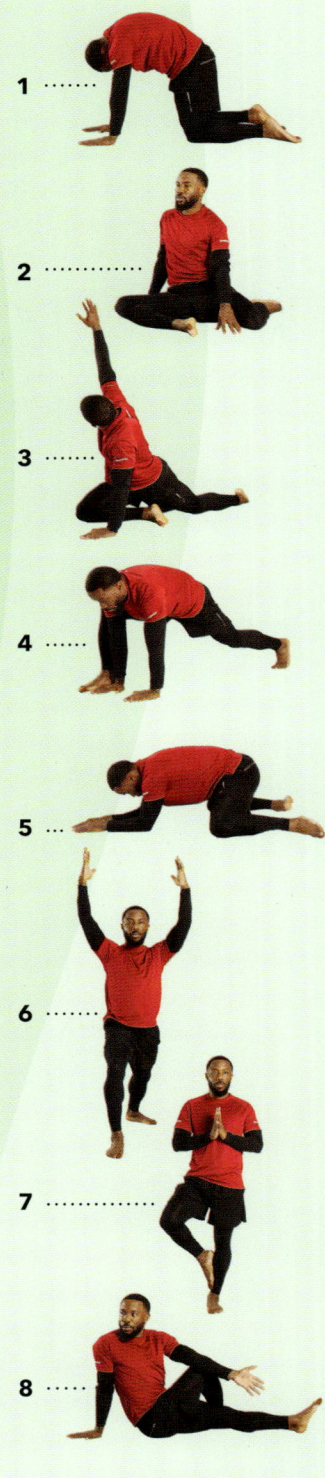

05 HIP ROUTINE

As a footballer, your hips and pelvis are exposed to an enormous amount of biomechanical stress, due to the continuous intensity of the game, so it's no surprise that football, especially if you've played from a young age, can lead to musculoskeletal changes and hence a decrease in the range of motion in the hips and surrounding areas, with the area most affected by injury being the groin.

Groin injuries are typically caused by sudden changes of direction, kicking, sprinting and high running load, all of which is what you do constantly during a game and for a lot of time on the training field. According to a 2021 article published in the *Joints* journal, these types of injuries, which produce pain in the lower abdominal, pubic or adductor areas, and can affect one side of the groin or both, make up between 8 and 18% of all football injuries. Of those groin injuries, 62% are adductor strains.

These muscular strains usually occur in your kicking leg, most commonly affecting the musculotendinous junction of the adductor longus or gracilis muscles, so integrating a hip routine or hip-focused postures is essential to prevent the muscle, tendon and ligaments strains and sprains that tend to cause groin pain.

A regular hip routine will also help prevent knee ligament injuries. By keeping the hips strong and balanced, especially the abductor (outer hip) muscles that play a crucial role in stabilising the pelvis, you help your knee to align correctly with your hips and ankles. Controlling the lower body and keeping it in alignment helps to decrease your susceptibility to anterior cruciate ligament (ACL) or medial collateral ligament (MCL) injuries.

The focus here is the hips, but the mixture of poses and movements in this routine not only promotes greater hip mobility, flexibility, strength and stability, but will also have a positive effect on the entire spine, upper and lower body, and help improve your overall performance on the pitch.

1 CAT AND COW

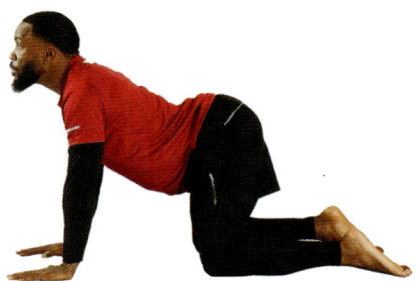 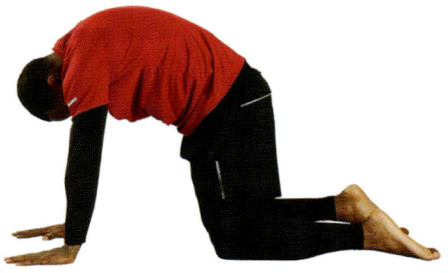

As you saw in the morning routine, cat and cow movements (see page 28) are great as a warm-up on their own or as part of the beginning of a routine because they stretch and mobilise the spine, creating space, and improving flexibility and circulation in the body. By supporting spinal health, they indirectly support better hip mobility which is essential for dynamic actions, such as sprinting, changing direction, rapid pivoting, tackling and kicking.

1. Begin on your hands and knees, in a tabletop position. Make sure your wrists, elbows and shoulders are in line, your knees are below your hips, hip-width apart, and your spine is in a neutral position, neither arched nor rounded.

2. As you inhale, drop your belly down, lift your head and chest up, and move your shoulders away from your ears (cow).

3. As you exhale, round your spine gently, bringing your chin towards your chest, as far as it feels comfortable (cat).

4. Take the length of a breath to move smoothly between these two poses and hold each pose for the length of a breath.

5. Repeat this flow of movement for several breaths, focusing on your breath and the movement of your spine. Imagine each vertebrae moves one at a time, starting from your tail bone and hips, moving up through your lower back, mid-back, neck and lastly your head.

2 90/90 WITH MOVEMENT

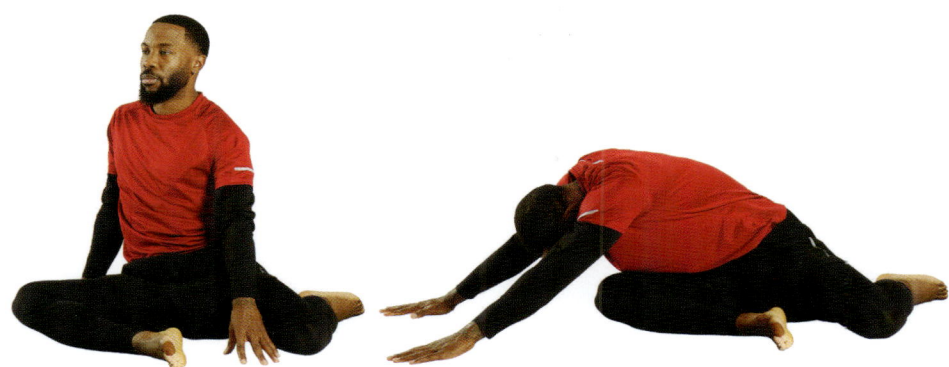

This is an excellent hip flexibility and mobility movement. It targets the internal and external rotation of the hips and stretches the glutes, hip flexors, lower back and surrounding muscles. The movement and sliding aspect of this pose helps to release the tension that builds up in the lower back, back of the hips and the outer hip muscles, helping you to develop the range of motion that is vital for efficient movement and the drive you need on the pitch.

1. Sit on the floor and bend your right leg at a 90-degree angle in front of your body with your hip rotated outward. Position it so your lower leg and knee are resting on the ground. Position your left leg at a 90-degree angle beside you with your hip rotated inward and your shin and ankle on the ground.

2. Stay in this position for a breath or two and notice what you're feeling where, in and around the hips.

3. Inhale and on your exhale start sliding your hands away from you in different directions. You can do short slides or long slides, so your trunk is parallel to the floor. There are no right or wrong movements when sliding your hands. Just move them to find out what you feel where, and to identify the tension and tight areas of your hips and lower back.

4. Slide your hands back.

5. Do these movements for a few deep and slow breaths or for as long as it feels good. Repeat on the other side.

3 PIGEON WITH TWISTS

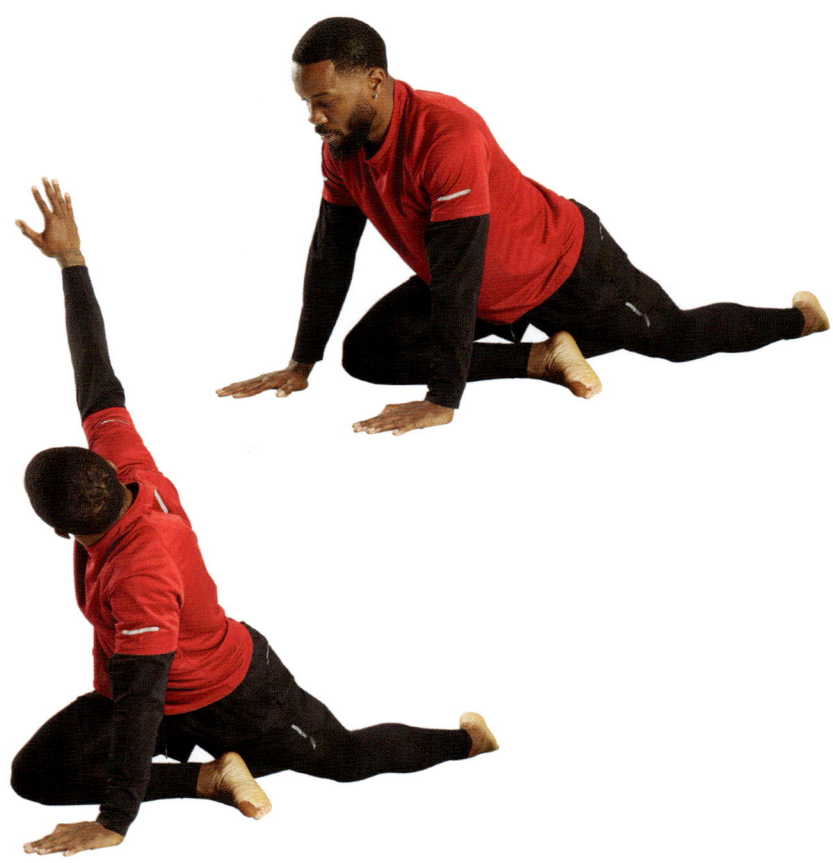

This pose is a powerful one for healthy hips. It deeply lengthens and releases tightness in the hip flexors, the outer hip and gluteus muscles, and having good flexibility in these muscles is key for maintaining good hip mobility.

The twist action added to this pose targets the spinal and lower back muscles, helping to ease tension and enhance overall flexibility, leading to muscle recovery, smooth movement on the pitch and reduced risk of injuries in those areas.

1. Begin on your hands and knees, in a tabletop position. Make sure your wrists, elbows and shoulders are in line, and your knees are below your hips, hip-width apart.

2. Inhale and on your exhale slide your right knee forward towards your right hand. Angle the lower part of your right foot so it is near your left hand.

3. Straighten and slide your left leg back, making sure the front of both hips

are in line and square. Place both hands on the floor or rest on your forearms, whatever feels most comfortable.

4. Inhale and as you exhale twist with your right arm and open towards the right. Slowly come back to the middle and on your next exhale twist with your left arm and open towards the left.

5. Repeat and alternate the twists for three to four rounds, breathing deeply and slowly as you move.

6. When you're done, slowly switch legs and repeat on the other side.

OPTIONAL PIGEON WITH TWISTS

You can also pause in the twists and hold them for a few deep and slow breaths, and you can deepen the pose by twisting to both sides with the same arm. So, for example, when you twist, open your right arm to your right. Then, when you come back to the middle, thread your right arm under your left arm and move it towards the left.

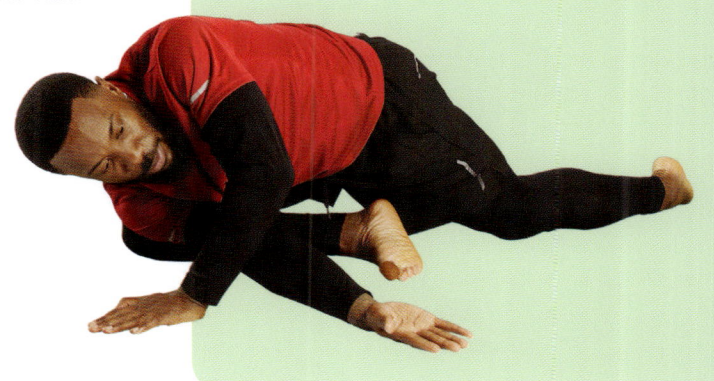

4 LIZARD

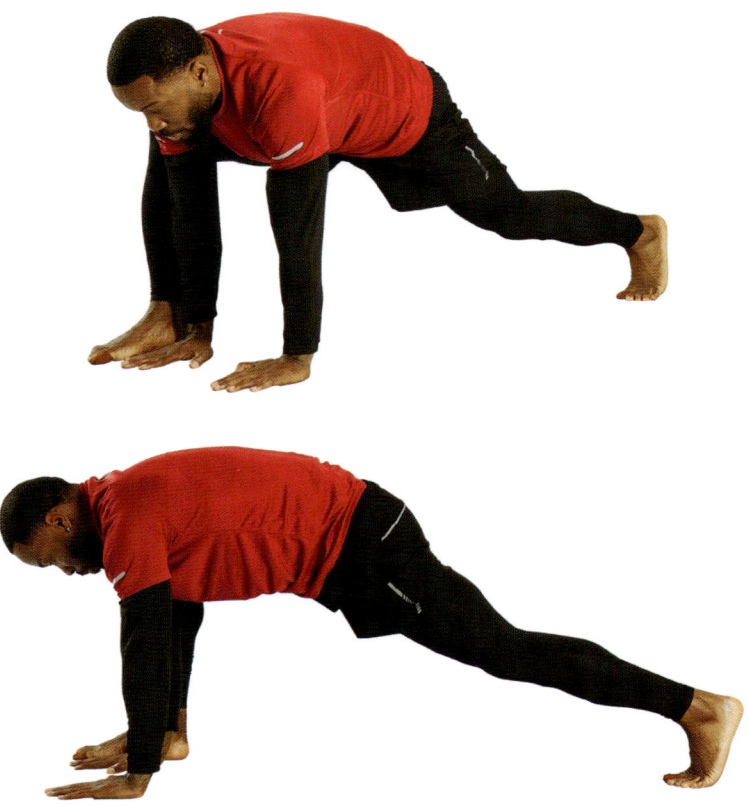

The lizard complements the other poses in this routine very well and together they can significantly improve your hip flexibility and mobility. This pose deeply lengthens the hip flexors and groin muscles, and depending on how tight your hamstrings are on the back leg you might feel a soft stretch there, too.

   This pose also engages the quads, glutes and core muscles, and helps to strengthen the muscles around the hip, leading to improved stability, balance and power during a game.

It strengthens shoulders, lengthens the abdominal muscles and can help lessen lower back pain or stiffness as well.

1. Begin on your hands and knees, in a tabletop position. Make sure your wrists, elbows and shoulders are in line, and your knees are below your hips, hip-width apart.

2. Inhale and on your exhale step your right foot forward and plant it on the outside of your right hand.

05 HIP ROUTINE

3. If your flexibility allows, on your next exhale lift your back knee off the floor. If it doesn't or you're totally new to this pose, keep your back knee on the floor.

4. Keep your arms straight, unless you're used to doing this pose with your forearms down and don't find it too intense.

5. As a variation you can add a twist to the pose by opening your right arm to the right side.

6. Hold the pose for five to eight breaths, focusing on deep and slow breaths.

7. To come out of the pose, if your knee is off the floor slowly lower it and then bring your right leg back into tabletop position. Take a breath and then repeat on the other side.

MODIFIED LIZARD

If the lizard is too intense for you, even with your arms straight and your back knee down, you may want to give the half happy baby a go. It is an effective hip opener, but offers a softer stretch.

It is the same position, but you lie on your back instead, with your arms beside your body, and legs straight and relaxed. Inhale and as you exhale bend one knee and bring it up to your chest, keeping your knee slightly to the side and in line with your armpit.

On your next exhale, either grab the outer edge of your foot, or the outside of your shin, or if still too intense sling a belt or long football sock over your foot, and bring the sole of your foot up facing the ceiling. Keep your other leg extended and hold the pose for five to eight breaths while focusing on deep and slow breaths.

When you're ready, slowly bring your leg back and plant your foot on the floor. Take a breath and then repeat on the other side.

5 FROG

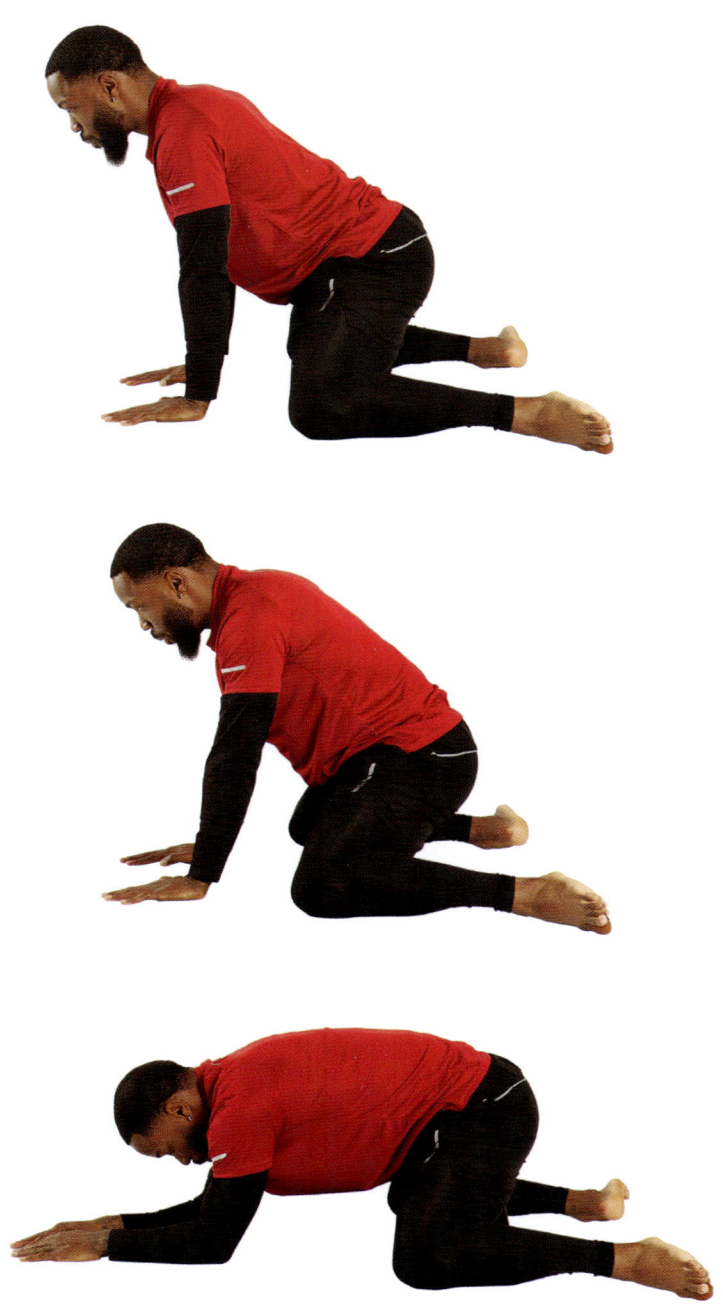

This pose focuses on the groin muscles (the adductors or inner thigh muscles). These muscles have to withstand a lot in football and hence this deep hip opener is highly beneficial for players.

The inner thighs often become tight due to the repetitive movements involved in football and hence groin injuries are at the top of the list of the most common footballing injuries. Working on range of motion and lengthening by improving the flexibility and mobility of the hips is therefore key.

Practising the frog regularly will help release tension, contributing to improved blood circulation, and promoting overall muscle recovery and relaxation. This leads to improved muscle balance function and better movement mechanics. Again, if you maintain healthy hips, you will reduce the risk of injuries, which should improve the longevity of your career.

NOTE
Remember that frog is a strong pose and you may feel some slight discomfort. However, you should not feel pain. Deep and slow breaths are important in this pose, so find a comfortable position where you can focus on your breathing, but still feel your muscles lengthening.

If you do feel discomfort in your knees, place a blanket under them for extra support. You may also want to place a couple of pillows or a bolster under your arms and upper body to make it easier to relax into the pose. This will make it more restorative and you can spend a little longer in it, two to three minutes perhaps, if it feels good for you. If you're new to this pose, you might want to take your time and slowly progress to longer holds.

1. Begin on your hands and knees, in the middle of your mat, facing the long side.

2. Inhale and as you exhale slowly widen and move your knees away from each other. The lower part of your legs should be parallel and your toes pointing outward.

3. On your next exhale gently lower your hips back and down towards the floor. Your hips and knees should be the same width apart.

4. Slowly lower your forearms to the floor, and focus on slow and deep breaths.

5. Hold the pose for four to eight deep and slow breaths, allowing yourself to relax a little bit more with each exhale.

6 WARRIOR 1

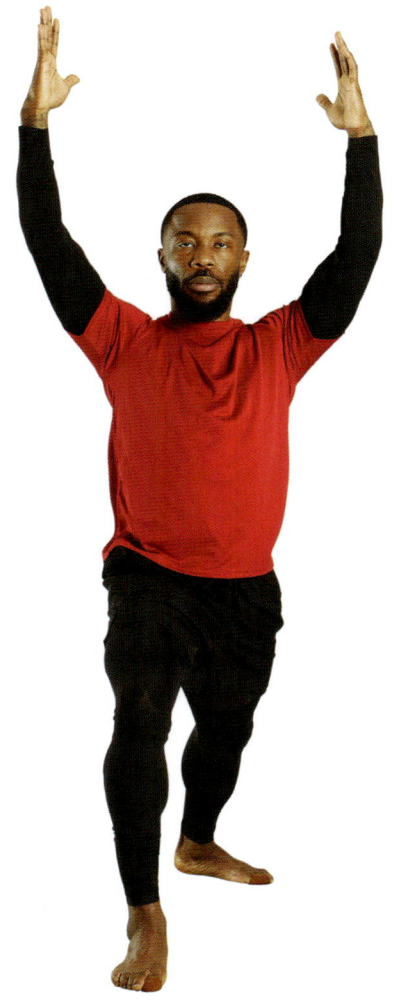

This powerful pose, just like a real warrior standing tall and ready for battle with inner strength, courage and focus, is so much more than 'just' a hip pose. Not only does it strengthen and stabilise your entire body, but it will also help you to foster the mental focus, endurance and confidence that symbolise a true warrior.

In warrior 1 (you may remember warrior 3 featured in the pre-training/pre-match routine – see page 53) the front knee is bent. This allows the quad muscles to strengthen, which helps to stabilise the knee, while the back leg is straight and engages the hamstring muscles to support the body and provide more stability. Maintaining

05 HIP ROUTINE

warrior 1 requires balance, but it also improves balance and the body's ability to stabilise itself by engaging the gluteus muscles in both the front and back leg.

In this position the groin muscles work to stabilise the pelvis and the muscles of the core, such as the rectus abdominis, obliques and erector spinae, helping stabilise the torso, and keeping the spine and back upright. The part where the arms are overhead involves and strengthens the upper body muscles as well, with the chest, shoulder and back muscles, such as the pectoralis major and minor, deltoids, trapezius and lats muscles, all engaged and working to raise and keep the arms overhead and the chest open.

1. Stand at the top of your mat with your feet hip-width apart.

2. Inhale and as you exhale step your left leg back (about a metre) until your front leg bends at the knee. Your left foot should turn out slightly, with your leg straight and strong.

3. Check your front knee to make sure that your right ankle and knee are in line, the middle of your right knee is in line with your second and third toes, and your right thigh is parallel to the floor.

4. Check the front bones of your hips are pointing forward and square.

5. Inhale and as you exhale lift your arms up and overhead, palms facing each other, shoulders down and relaxed. Gaze forward. Draw your belly button gently in towards your spine to keep your core active.

6. Hold this position for five to eight breaths, while focusing on deep and slow breaths.

7. Slowly return your back leg to the front of the mat. Pause for a breath then repeat on the other side.

NOTE
If five to eight breaths are too many, start with what feels best for you and then progress. Similarly, if it is too much of a stretch with your arms up you can leave your arms beside your body at first and then, as your hips and legs become more flexible, incorporate raised arms.

7 TREE

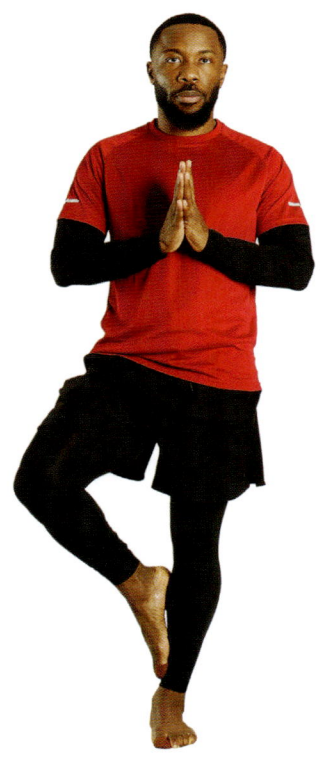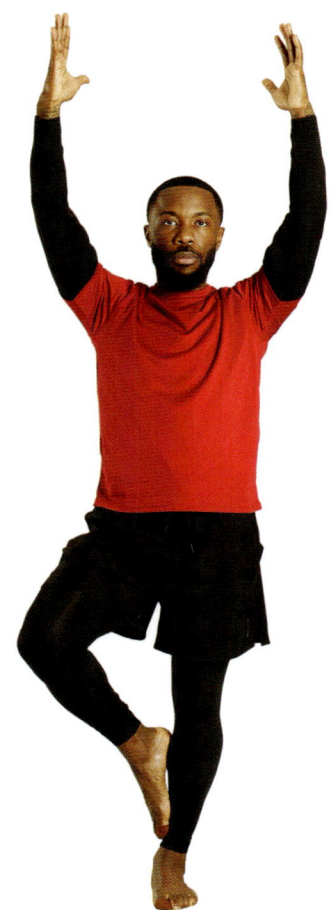

This pose is not only excellent for hip health, but it also benefits the entire lower body and core. It strengthens the muscles of the standing leg, particularly targeting the outer hip muscles (abductors), which are crucial for stabilising the hips, and maintaining form and alignment in the lower body.

Tree also strengthens the quadriceps, calves and ankle stabilisers of the standing leg, which are essential for improving stability and providing the strength needed for jumping and maintaining control when landing.

Additionally, it activates the core muscles, improving the distribution of power throughout the body.

Among the benefits of this pose is that it enhances the range of motion of the lifted leg, gently opening up the hips and lengthening the adductors (groin) muscles, which once more enhances flexibility. Since this pose is performed on one side at a time, it is superb for promoting balance symmetry and helps correct any muscle imbalances.

05 HIP ROUTINE

1. Stand with your feet hip-width apart. Lengthen your spine and keep your hips in neutral, so your tail bone is pointing down.

2. Inhale and as you exhale shift all your weight on to your left foot. Lift your right foot and, with your toes pointing down, position the sole of your foot inside your shin, or at the top of your left leg, against your groin.

3. Keep your hips square. Focus on a point in front of you and feel your engaged core.

4. Bring your palms together and place them in front of your chest, thumbs touching your sternum.

5. Focus on deep and slow breaths. If your foot is against your groin, press it into your groin and your groin into your foot. Hold the pose for 15 to 60 seconds.

6. For added balance, extend your arms above your head, keeping them wider than shoulder-width apart, and making sure your shoulders are relaxed and down.

7. To come out of the pose, slowly lower your right foot to the floor. Shake the standing leg and ankle, then repeat on the other side.

NOTE
Never position your foot on the inside of your knee. If you can't place it against your groin, start by placing it on the inside of the opposite foot or inside your shin, but never on your knee. Make sure your hips stay in neutral, continue to point forward and are square, and check your pelvis isn't tilting.

8 HALF LORD OF THE FISH

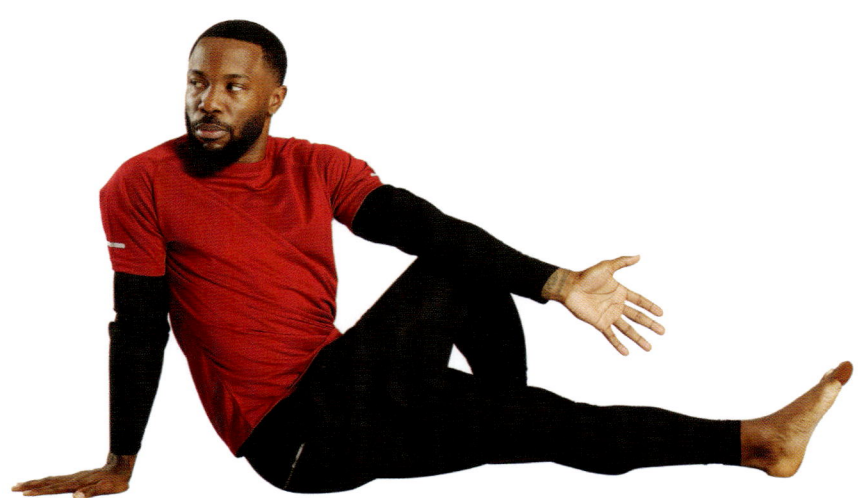

As you have probably noticed by now, a flexible spine is the way to maintain happy and healthy hips. This pose works predominantly on improving the flexibility and mobility of the spine by providing a deep spinal twist and a profound stretch of the gluteus, the outer hip and the deep hip rotator muscles.

Including this pose regularly into your practice will help to ease muscular tension and tightness in the hips, which is very common in footballers. Less tension in the hips leads to more efficient and powerful movements on the pitch.

The half lord of the fish also supports balanced muscle function and alignment, which is essential for maintaining proper posture and movement mechanics, and in turn is key for enhancing performance and making sure that the movement is carried out in the most effective way.

05 HIP ROUTINE

1. Sit in the middle of your mat and with your legs straight out in front of you.

2. Keep your left leg extended and bend your right leg, placing your right foot on the outside of your left hip.

3. As you inhale, keep your spine upright and as you exhale twist your torso to the right, placing your right hand on the floor behind you.

4. On your next exhale, if your mobility allows, place your left elbow on the outside of your right knee and deepen the twist. If your mobility doesn't allow you to reach the outside of your knee with your elbow, hug your knee or leg instead.

5. Hold the pose for five to eight breaths, focusing on slow and deep breaths. With each exhale you may want to deepen the twist.

6. Slowly come back to the middle and do a brief counter twist to your left, then repeat on the other side.

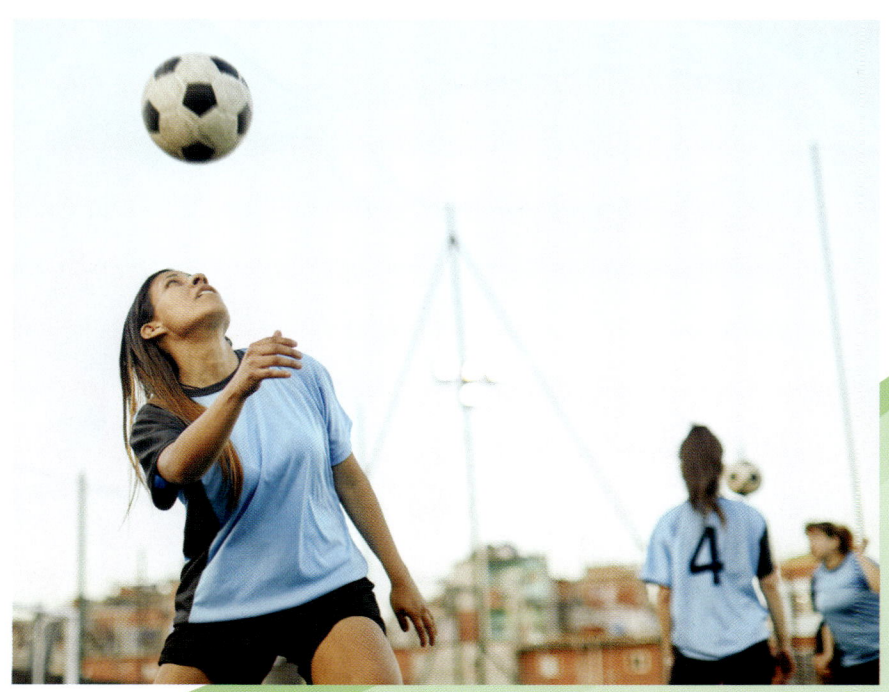

06 HAMSTRING ROUTINE

1. The extender .... page 104
2. Namaste .... page 106
3. Pyramid .... page 108
4. Wide-legged forward bend with twists .... page 110
5. Standing forward bend with twists .... page 112
6. Half split (toes up and down) .... page 114
7. Hamstring strap stretch .. page 116

Hamstring injuries are very common among footballers and all too frequently they come back time and time again.

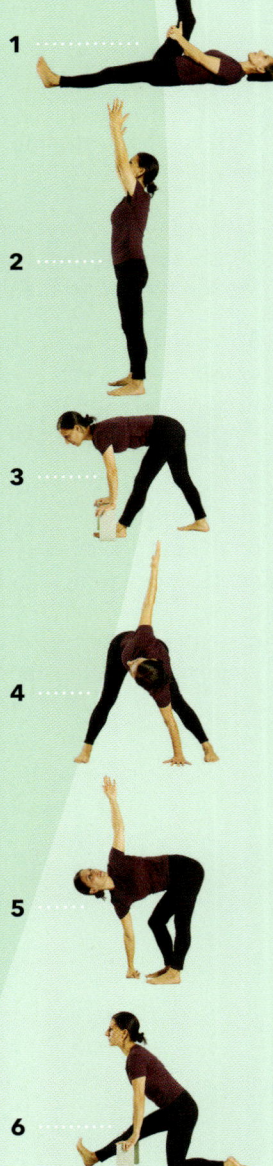

06 HAMSTRING ROUTINE

In a professional team of 25 players, about five of them will suffer hamstring injuries every season. That's around 80 days of lost football. Hamstring injuries are one of the most common injuries in football and they are usually triggered by sprinting, stretching, a combination of both, or overuse. The results can be strains, ruptures, tears and inflammation in the belly of the muscle, within the tissue at the top or bottom of the back of the thigh, or in the actual tendon itself.

Unfortunately, the recurrence of this type of injury is also high, probably because players are called back to play too soon or because rehabilitation programmes are ineffective. In most cases, when an injury takes place, and once a player is fully rehabbed and has returned to playing, there is still a window of 12 months, or sometimes longer, where the risk of a re-injury to the same site is high.

Depending on the type of injury, severity and how long the player was out for, the risk of a new injury to the area above or below the initial injury is also common. Therefore, it is important to continue to rehab and prehab, do the extra work and integrate the right kind of exercises into your routine.

This hamstring routine consists of a combination of yoga poses and other exercises that I have found very helpful for players as a part of their prehab and rehab protocols, and which are primarily designed to support the lengthening of your hamstring muscle-tendon unit. The lengthening action helps enhance your hamstring muscle motion, so the muscle and tendon tissue becomes stronger, more flexible, better able to deal with impact and more resilient to injury.

1 THE EXTENDER

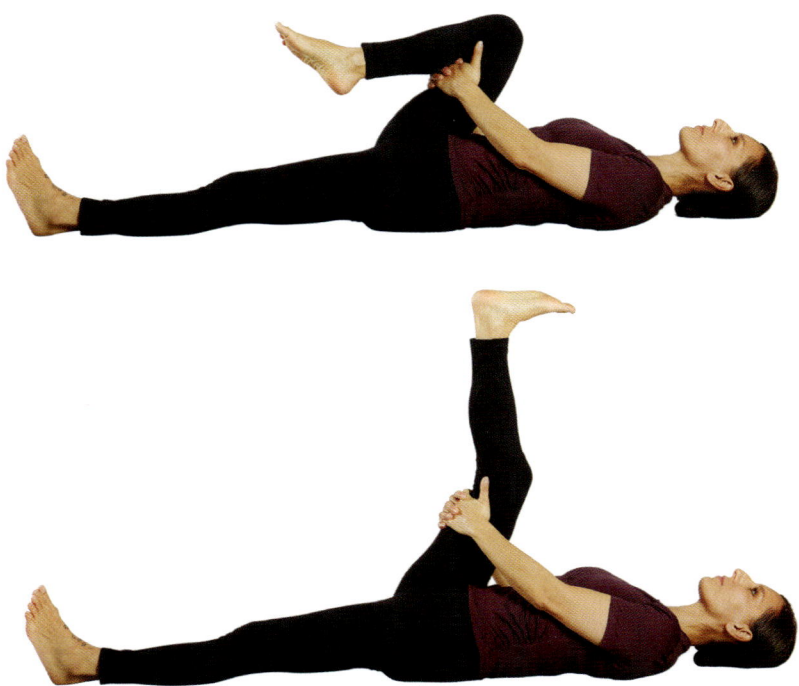

The extender is a hamstring rehabilitation exercise that is part of the Askling L-Protocol, which focuses on the eccentric loading (when a muscle lengthens under pressure) of the hamstring muscles and aims to accelerate a player's return to full play. This exercise was created for players coming back from different types of acute hamstring injuries and has been found to be more effective than conventional hamstring rehab exercises. In a study in the *American Journal of Sports Medicine*, participants in the Askling L-Protocol group using eccentric exercises, including the extender, had quicker recovery times and a lower re-injury rate compared to those following traditional rehabilitation methods.

Although the extender is primarily used for rehabilitation, it can also help with injury prevention, and I recommend it for both rehabilitation and prevention, particularly if you have had previous hamstring injuries or occasionally experience discomfort in your hamstrings. I suggest performing it on both legs.

06 HAMSTRING ROUTINE

1. Lie on your back, flex your hip, bring your right leg up to 90 degrees and hold it with both hands.

2. Inhale and on the exhale, straighten your leg as much as you can without feeling any pain in your hamstring.

3. Pause for a couple of seconds at the top with your leg extended, then slowly start bending your leg at the knee and allowing your heel to drop.

4. Repeat on the other side.

5. For rehab purposes, repeat this exercise for three sets of twelve repetitions and perform it twice a day. For prehab purposes, repeat this exercise for two to three sets of ten to twelve repetitions, as part of your warm-up routine, two to three times a week.

NOTE
When doing this movement, rather than thinking that the knee bends and extends, imagine that the heel drives the movement away from the body and then back down. This will make the movement smoother. To progress you may increase the speed when straightening your leg.

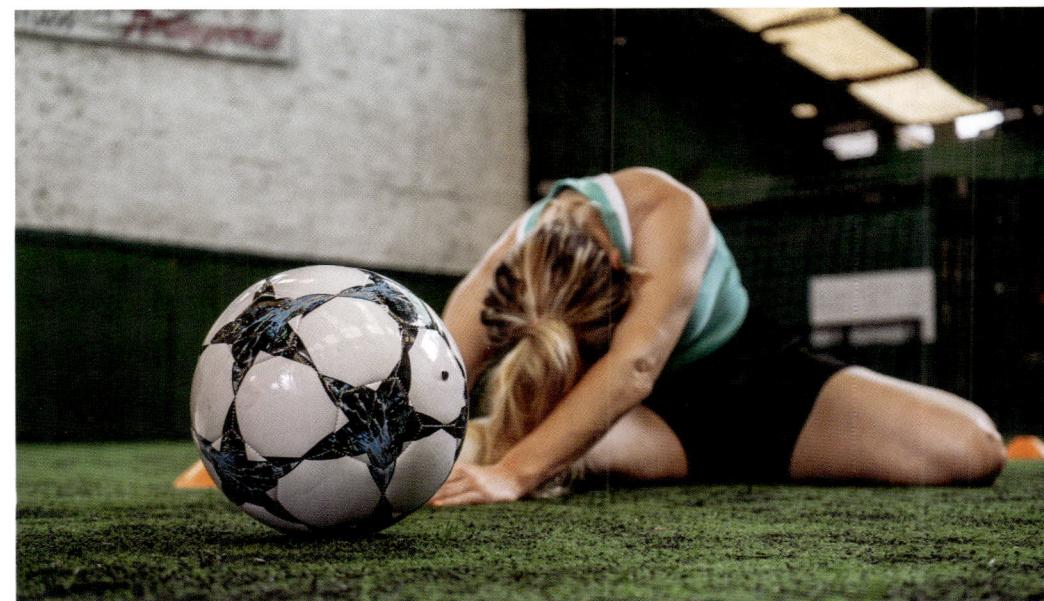

2 NAMASTE

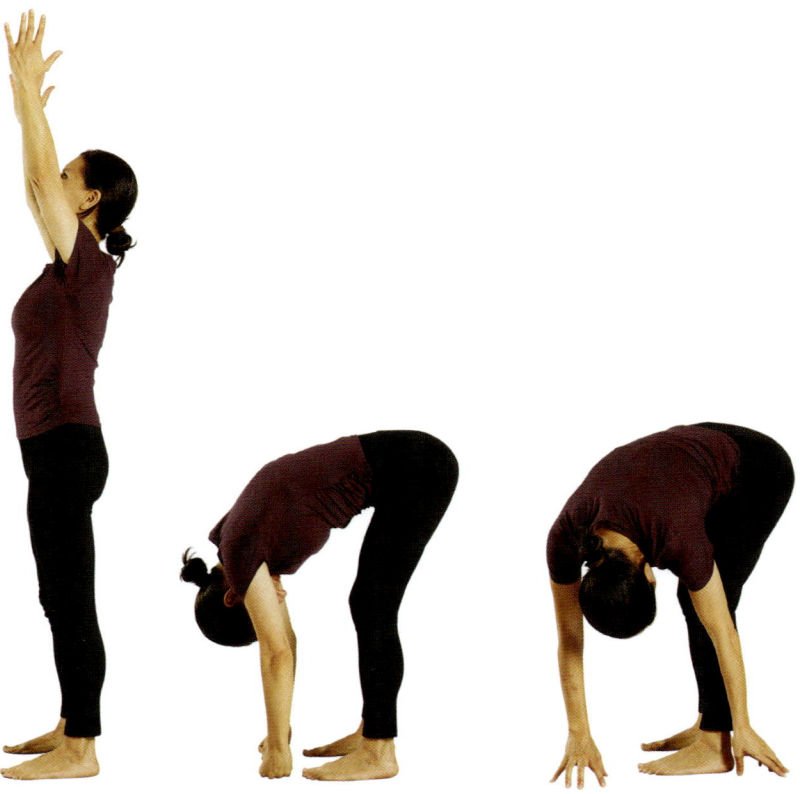

If you have tried the morning routine (see page 36) and the pre-training/pre-match routine (see page 42), you will already be familiar with namaste. It has a range of benefits, and if your calves and hamstrings are tight, you will feel them too being stretched as you fold forward.

While in your forward bend, with your fingers touching the floor, since your head is below your heart, blood flow to your brain is enhanced and you will therefore feel very peaceful, but also energised, because of the increased flow of oxygen to your muscles and organs.

As you move from side to side, you will feel the side of your body and your hips opening up, enhancing flexibility and lengthening in those areas. This full movement releases stress, anxiety and fatigue, and is great to perform whenever you feel it will be beneficial, but it is particularly effective for lengthening of the posterior line of the body.

06 HAMSTRING ROUTINE

1. Stand with your feet hip-width apart and your arms at your sides. Be aware of your posture, stand tall and tuck your shoulder blades in slightly.

2. As you inhale, open up your chest and lift your arms up towards the ceiling, gently arching your back as you look up towards your hands. These can be facing each other or your palms can be touching.

3. As you exhale, bring your hands down through the midline of your body and, with your chin tucked in to your chest, slowly move them towards the floor and bend forwards.

4. Releasing your hands, allow your fingers to touch the floor. If your fingers don't touch the floor, bend your knees slightly. You might also need to bend your knees if your hamstrings are very tight, but if so, do make sure your hips are still as high as possible.

5. Bend forward, with at least your fingertips touching the floor and your head heavy.

6. Move your hips from side to side, allowing your fingers to draw semi-circles, for a breath or two.

7. When you feel ready to come up, keep your chin near your chest and slowly roll up, with your head coming up last. As you open your chest, lift your arms up towards the sky and look up towards your hands again. That is one round.

8. Continue this flow for five to six rounds or until you feel loosened up, making sure you breathe deeply throughout the movement.

3 PYRAMID

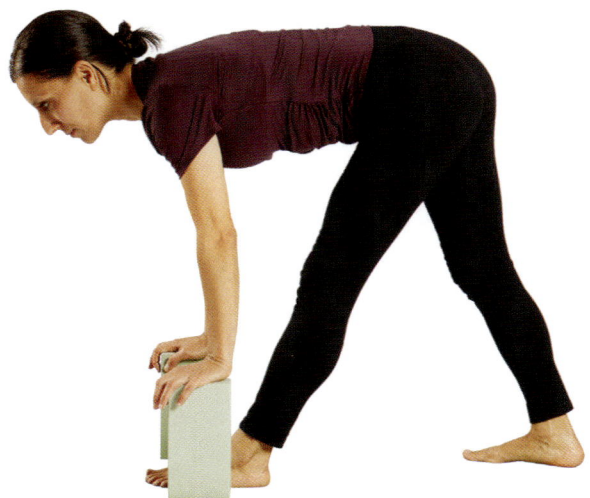

A deep stretch that helps to lengthen the hamstrings, calves, Achilles tendon and back of the hip muscles, pyramid also aligns and opens the hips, enhancing overall hip mobility. It adds a soft stretch to the spine, too, supporting better posture and helping to lower the risk of lower back injuries.

By including this pose regularly in your weekly prehab routines, you can, over time, reduce the risk of imbalances and therefore be less prone to hamstring injuries. The improved range of motion will have a positive effect on your performance, especially your stride length, speed, agility and kicking power. Like the other poses in this routine, this one is also great for optimising recovery, and reducing muscle soreness and tightness.

1. Stand with your feet hip-width apart. If positioning your feet wider than hip-width apart feels more comfortable for you then perform it that way, but make sure your stance is not too narrow.

2. Inhale and on the exhale step your right foot back (about one foot), with your toes pointing slightly out to the side. Keep your hips pointing forwards and square.

3. Inhale and lengthen your spine. On your exhale press your hips slightly back and lean your upper body forward as far as is comfortable. Keep your head in line with your spine and your back flat as you lower yourself, bringing your trunk towards the front of your thighs.

4. Once you have bent forward as far as feels comfortable, you can relax your head and slightly round your upper spine. Bend your knees slightly if you want to, and rest your fingers and hands on the floor, or on blocks or books, on either side of your front foot.

5. Keep your eyes slightly in front of you or on your shins if this feels more comfortable for your neck.

6. Hold this pose for 15 to 30 seconds, focusing on slow and deep breaths.

7. Once you get into a habit of doing this pose regularly, you can also focus on lengthening your spine with each inhale and taking the forward bend a little deeper with each exhale.

8. To come out of the pose, gently bend both knees and slowly come up. Repeat on the other side.

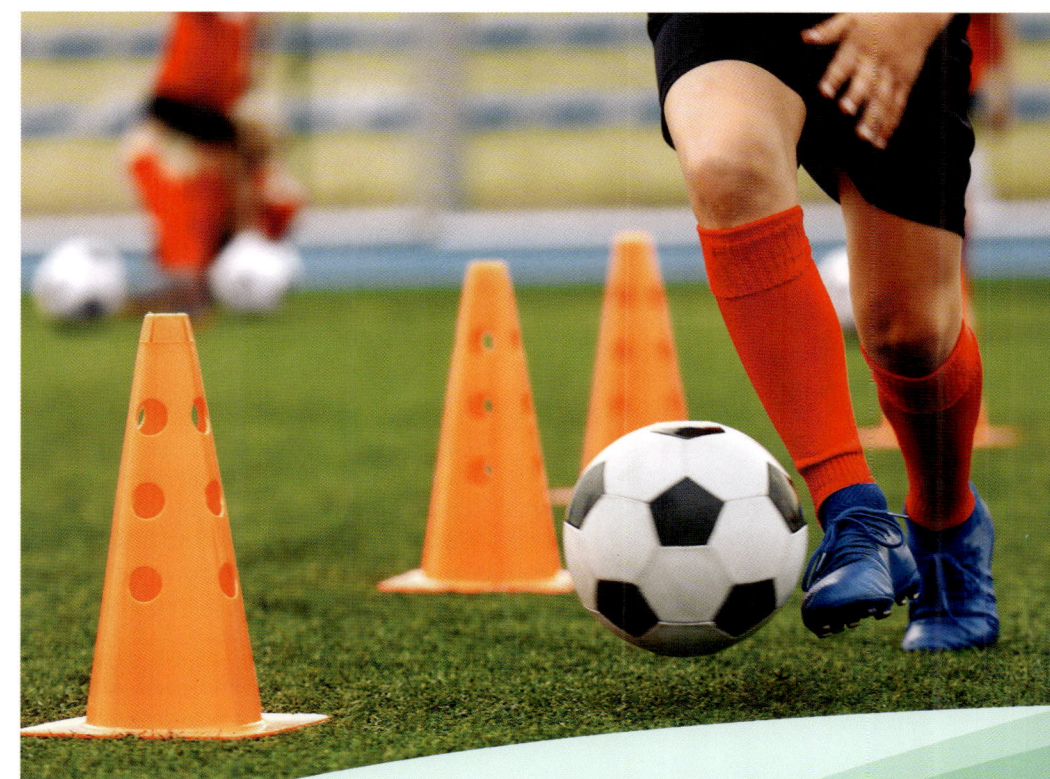

YOGA FOR FOOTBALLERS

4. WIDE-LEGGED FORWARD BEND WITH TWISTS

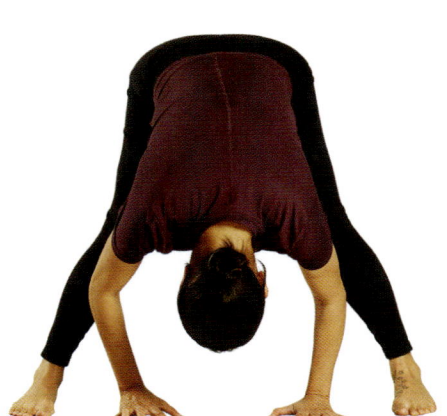
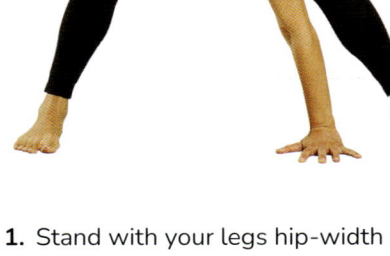

This pose has many great benefits for footballers, especially as a part of a hamstring prehab routine. This wide-legged forward bend offers a deep stretch for the hamstrings and inner thigh muscles, and helps to improve the length of the hamstrings and overall hip flexibility. This will lead to better explosive moments and more efficient movement patterns on the pitch.

The twisting motion improves spinal mobility and supports good spinal health, while strengthening the core muscles, which helps to maintain stability and balance – crucial for the coordination and quick changes of direction required in football.

1. Stand with your legs hip-width apart.

2. Inhale and bring your arms out to the side and up above your head.

3. Exhale and fold forward, keeping a slight bend in your knees so your fingers can reach the floor.

4. In your forward bend start moving your feet further apart. Make sure the position is comfortable, but from the front your body should look like a pyramid or an upside-down letter V. If your groin muscles are very tight you will feel them here.

5. Allow your head to be heavy and hang, looking on the floor behind you.

6. Stay in this wide-legged forward bend for a breath or two, feeling how the hamstrings and the groin muscles are lengthening and strengthening.

7. Keeping your hips square and your left hand on the floor, inhale and on the exhale twist and open your right chest, arm and side of your face to the right.

8. Hold the twist for the full exhale or another breath or two, before slowly coming back to the middle, and allowing your head to relax and be heavy again.

9. Repeat the twist on the left side.

10. Alternate the twists with either a pause at each end, just the movement or a mixture of movement and pause, for five to six repetitions or as many as feels good.

NOTE
When you are adding the twists, think about them in terms of the chest opening up first, followed by an extension of the arm and then the head turning, rather than the arm leading the twist.

5. STANDING FORWARD BEND WITH TWISTS

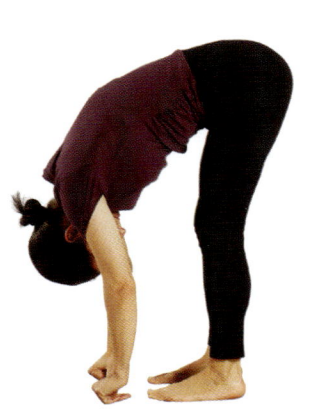
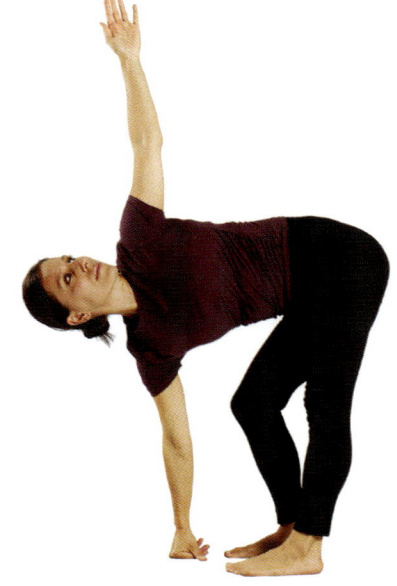

This pose is very similar to the wide-legged forward bend with twists, both in terms of the movements and the benefits. Here we are still working on the flexibility of the hamstring and calf muscles, and spinal mobility, but since we have the legs hip-width apart, instead of the adductors, we are working on lengthening the outer hip muscles, the abductors.

The latter muscles play a fundamental role in stabilising the pelvis, hip and knee joint. Good flexibility in those muscles is key to facilitating wide, lateral movements and improving agility, so when you change directions, you aren't just quick but smooth, too. More power can also be generated when these muscles are not overly tight and are regularly being lengthened.

1. Stand with your legs hip-width apart.

2. Inhale and bring your arms out to the side and up above your head.

3. Exhale and fold forward, keeping a slight bend in your knees so your fingers can reach the floor.

4. Stay in your forward bend for a breath or two.

5. Inhale and on the exhale bend your right knee.

6. Place the fingers of your right hand, or your whole hand, on the floor. Inhale and on the exhale twist and open your left chest, arm and side of your face towards the left, keeping your left leg straight and your hips square.

06 HAMSTRING ROUTINE

7. Hold the twist for the full exhale or another breath or two, before slowly coming back to the middle, and allowing your head to relax and be heavy again.

8. Repeat the twist on the right side.

9. Alternate the twists with either a pause at each end, just the movement or a mixture of movement and pause, for five to six repetitions or as many as feels good.

NOTE
When performing the twist, if you're very new to this movement or feel a lot of tension in your legs, bend both your legs at the knee slightly. Otherwise, keep one knee bent and the other one (on the side you're twisting towards) straight. This will deepen the stretch and allow more lengthening in the hamstrings and outer hips on that side. To get deeply into lengthening the abductors you will need to add the twist and keep the leg you're twisting towards straight.

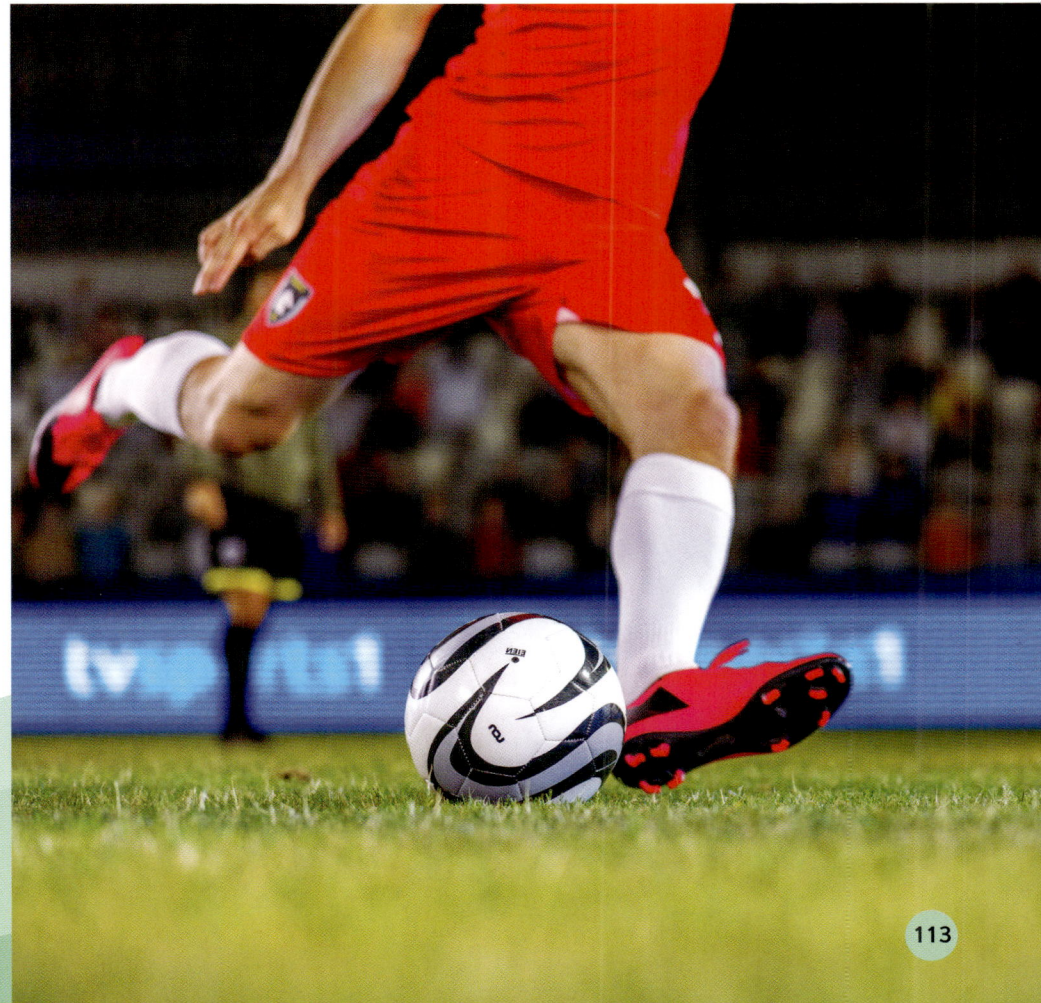

6 HALF SPLIT (TOES UP AND DOWN)

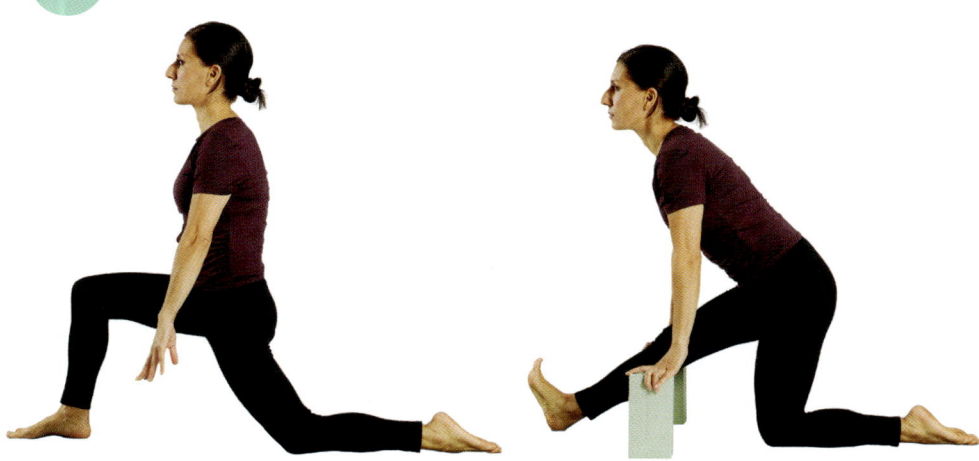

It appears in the post-training/post-match routine (see page 64), but the half split is included here, too, because it's very beneficial for the overall health of your hamstrings, calves and ankles. It offers a strong stretch for the hamstrings and helps to maintain good muscle length, and hence decreases the risk of some of the most common injuries to the back of the leg, such as strains and tears.

This pose is usually performed with the toes pointing up, which is great since it targets the calf muscles and Achilles tendon, and helps to lengthen these areas. However, by moving your toes down as well, and keeping your foot planted on the floor, it really helps footballers strengthen and improve the flexibility of their ankle joints, leading to an enhanced range of motion and better overall stability, which will help prevent ankle injuries, such as sprains.

1. Start in a low lunge position with your left knee on the mat and right leg forward, your ankle and knee in one line. Keep your hips square.

2. Inhale and as you exhale, shift your hips back and straighten your right leg, with your fingers touching the mat, or resting on the blocks, on either side of your front leg.

3. Inhale and flex the toes of your right foot up towards the ceiling. As you exhale, point them down to the floor. The backs of your toes might not touch the mat initially.

4. Once you have moved your toes up and down a few times, keep them pointing upwards, exhale and lean your upper body forward over your right leg. Make sure your spine is nice and long, and your head is in line with your spine.

5. Stay here for a couple of breaths. If you want to deepen the stretch on the back of the hamstring, flex your foot a little more.

6. Inhale and on the exhale slowly move back to the initial low lunge position, placing your hands on either side of your hips.

06 HAMSTRING ROUTINE

7. Engage your core muscles by gently squeezing your belly button towards your spine, keeping your upper body upright, shoulders stacked in line with your hips and your tail bone pointing down towards the floor to maintain a straight line through your spine.

8. Inhale and on your exhale very gently lean your chest and upper body back, without creating too much of a curve in your lower back. Hold this pose for two to three breaths or as long as it feels good.

9. Slowly release and repeat on the other side.

NOTE
If you're new to this, and/or very tight at the front of your ankle, it can initially be a bit uncomfortable to point your toes down to the floor.

You can place blocks or books on either side of you for extra support, or if your hands do not reach the floor. If you have knee issues, you can also fold a blanket and place it under your knee for extra comfort and support.

When in the lunge position, keep your tail bone pointing down towards the floor, so your hips are in neutral, not tilting forwards or backwards, which can sometimes happen. This helps avoid unnecessary strain on the hips and lower back, and also aids engagement of the lower abdominal muscles.

OPTION
While you are here, you may want to deepen the low lunge, and get more into the hips and hip flexors, by adding arm variations. For example, instead of placing your hands on your hips, reach your arms overhead, with your shoulders relaxed and away from your ears, shoulder blades slightly tucked in and palms facing each other. Alternatively, you can raise your arms above your head and hold on to opposite forearms, or interlock your hands placed behind your head. Whichever position you choose, gently lean the back of your head into either your arms or hands.

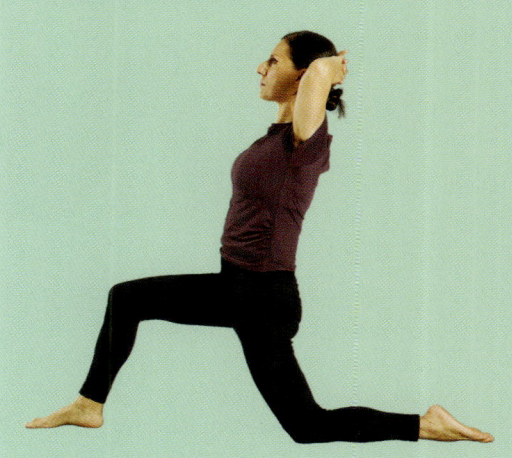

7 HAMSTRING STRAP STRETCH

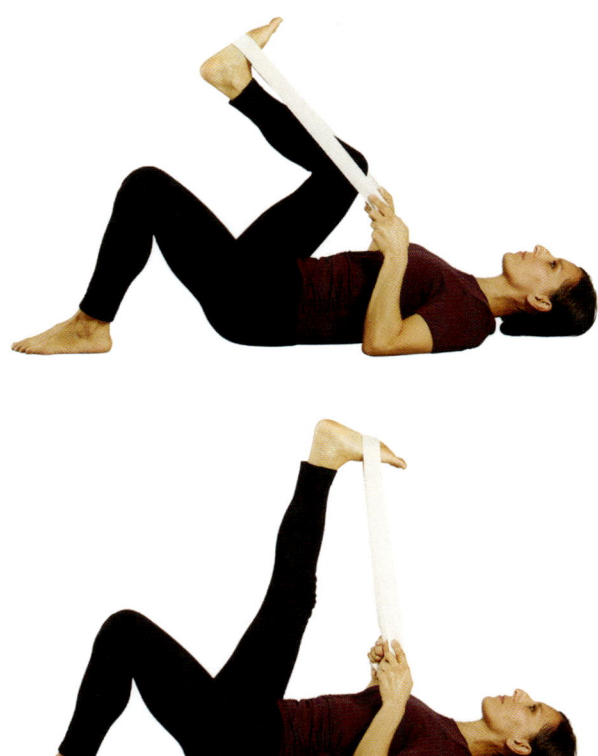

The hamstring strap stretch is great to practise when you have tight hamstrings and really need to have a good stretch, yet you're feeling tired and just want to lie down. It's particularly effective for maintaining hamstring muscle elasticity, allowing you to quickly accelerate and decelerate when making quick manoeuvres on the pitch.

This pose is not only great for improving the flexibility of the hamstrings, but also for the entire posterior chain – the group of muscles that run from your feet to your neck, up the back of your body, including your lower back, glutes and calf muscles – especially when the toes are fully flexed down. Having this greater flexibility in the posterior chain, for example, is one way of helping your calves avoid getting cramp in the last 20 minutes of a game.

If your opposite leg is extended and down on the floor, and your hip flexors are tight, you will feel a nice relief in that area, too. This improved range of motion will allow you to move with more fluidity on the pitch.

06 HAMSTRING ROUTINE

1. Lie on your back with your feet on the floor, and your knees bent and pointing up towards the ceiling.

2. Bring your right foot up and loop the strap around the arch.

3. Inhale and on your exhale extend your right leg up towards the ceiling as much as possible, keeping your right knee slightly bent if needed and your toes pointing down towards you.

4. Fully inhale and exhale, and find the position where you're most comfortable. Hold the strap with both hands, and keep your head and back of your upper body resting on the floor. Your left leg, which is on the floor, can be kept bent or straightened.

5. Focus on deep and slow breaths, holding the pose for 30 seconds.

6. Slowly bend your right leg and remove the strap. Repeat on the other side.

NOTE
If you haven't got a strap, you can use a belt or a long football sock. Another way of doing this exercise is to use a wall near a doorway, placing one leg on the wall and the other through the door.

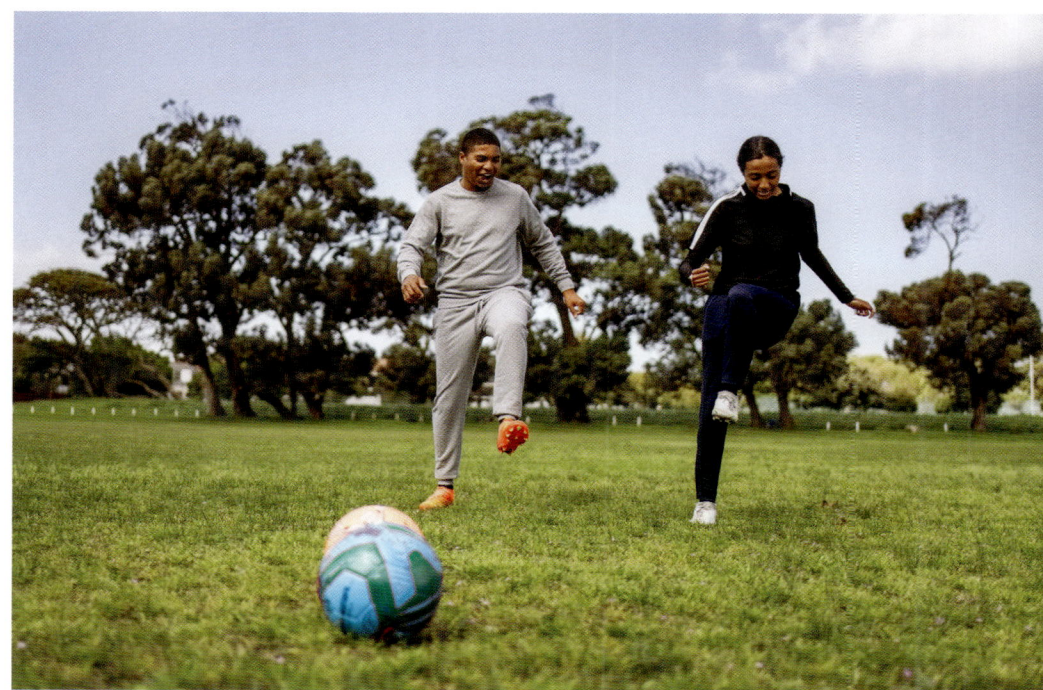

07 LOWER BACK ROUTINE

1. Spinal dance .... page 120
2. Thread the needle .... page 121
3. Low lunge cactus arms .... page 123
4. Bridge .... page 124
5. Rock 'n' rolls .... page 126
6. Locust .... page 127
7. Reversed tabletop .... page 128
8. Cobra press-ups .... page 129
9. Child's pose to cobra flow .... page 130

Many footballers experience acute lower back injuries during training sessions or matches, and many also develop chronic lower back problems.

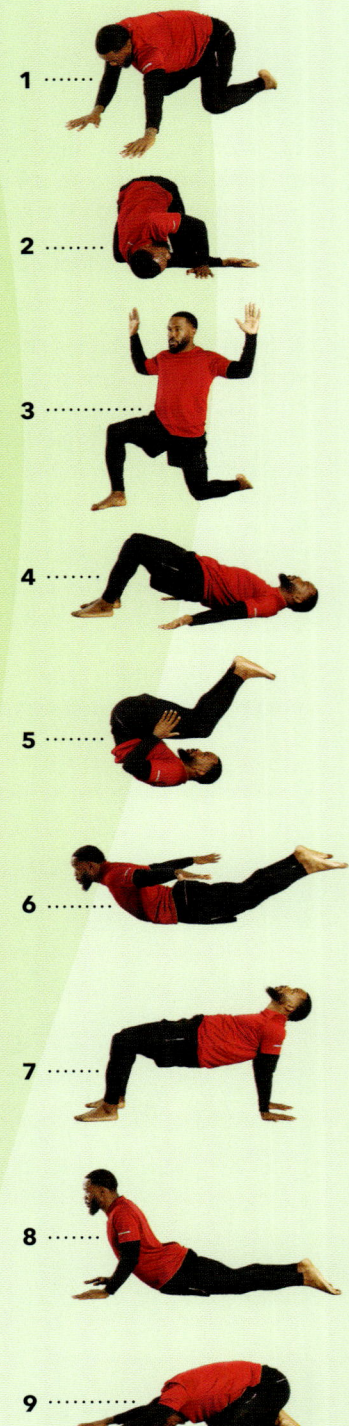

07 LOWER BACK ROUTINE

Lower back issues are very common among footballers. The nature of the sport, combined with the hours of training and games, and the unique physical manoeuvres on the pitch, imposes significant mechanical loads on the spine, particularly compressive forces on the lumbar region. This creates a clear link between the physical demands of the sport and injury risk.

The amount of time spent on the pitch and in the gym, combined with high training intensity, often without adequate recovery, leads to tissue overload, recurrent injuries and chronic lower back problems. Younger players are particularly at risk due to their still-developing musculoskeletal systems, which are more vulnerable to skeletal damage and structural abnormalities under stress.

There are also the many hours of travel, both pre- and post-match, regardless of the league or level of play, but especially for away games. Prolonged periods of sitting during coach, train or plane travel again place additional compressive forces on the spine, aggravating discomfort and pain in the lower back.

During certain parts of the season, some clubs also play European midweek fixtures on top of their regular weekly league games, often flying back immediately after matches. Sitting on an airplane post-match is particularly detrimental to recovery. The decreased atmospheric pressure impairs muscle recovery, reduces blood flow and circulation, and slows down the metabolism of lactic acid. This can result in increased stiffness in the body, especially in the lower back and hips.

All these factors contribute to why so many footballers suffer from chronic and recurrent lower back issues, often leading to early degenerative joint disease. This is why it is essential to incorporate exercises like those that follow into your training regimen. The poses and movements in this routine will help decrease muscle tension, improve blood flow and circulation, and allow you to better manage lower back issues, while reducing injury risk, maintaining performance and keeping your lumbar spine healthy.

1 SPINAL DANCE

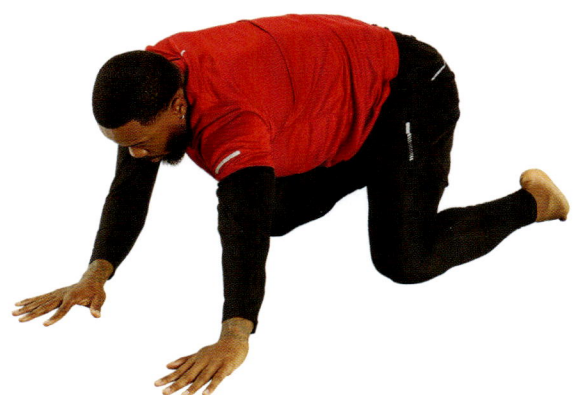

Ideal for releasing tension and loosening up the hips, pelvis, lower back and spine, you may have noticed that spinal dance is also in the post-training/post-match routine (see page 60) because players often experience tightness in their lower back and hips due to the physical demands of their game or training. This simple movement increases the blood flow to these problem areas, helping to improve hip and spinal flexibility and mobility, and hence aid lower back pain relief.

1. Begin on your hands and knees, in a tabletop position. Make sure your wrists, elbows and shoulders are in line, and your knees are below your hips, hip-width apart.

2. Inhale and on the exhale slowly start to move your hips in a circular movement.

3. You can switch between moving clockwise and anticlockwise, and making smaller and bigger circles – whatever feels good and comfortable for you – but create a fluid and smooth movement, with no beginning or end, and focus on your inhales and exhales, breathing deeply and slowly.

4. Move for a few breaths, until you feel your hips and back are starting to loosen up, and your body feels warmer.

5. You can perform this movement for one or a few rounds, shaking your wrists out a little between rounds if you want to.

OPTIONAL SPINAL DANCE

Combining spinal dance with cat and cow (see page 28) can be very effective, so try moving your hips for a few rounds then adding a couple of rounds or more of cat and cow, before going back to your hips, and so on. It is also beneficial to add a few rounds of shoulder circles to release the tension in your upper back and chest muscles, while improving your shoulder mobility.

07 LOWER BACK ROUTINE

2   THREAD THE NEEDLE

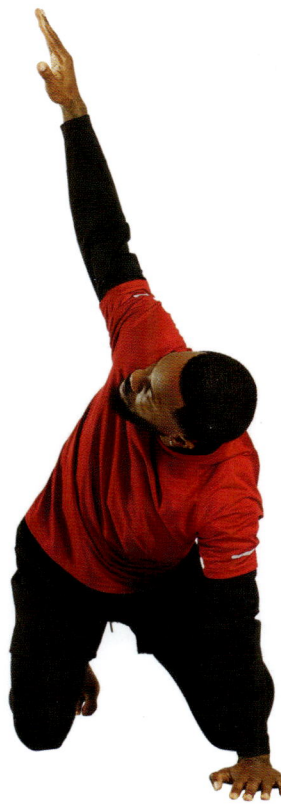
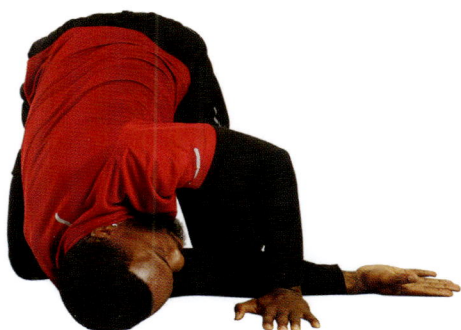

As a follow-up to spinal dance this is excellent, as it complements it very well. Thread the needle is specifically included here as a warm-up and to open up, stretch and alleviate tightness in the spine, hips and shoulders, and hence give relief to any discomfort in the lower back while improving overall flexibility in all those areas.

1. Begin on your hands and knees, in a tabletop position. Make sure your wrists, elbows and shoulders are in line, and your knees are below your hips, hip-width apart.

2. Inhale and on the exhale lift and open the right side of your chest and then your right arm as far as is comfortable, followed by your head. Look towards your right arm or that side of the room.

continues overleaf

3. Inhale and on the exhale scoop your right arm through the left one, lowering your right shoulder and the right side of your head towards the floor. Allow your face to rest on the mat if that feels comfortable and your mobility allows. If it doesn't, go as far as feels good for you.

4. Make sure your left hand is active and pressing into the floor, and your wrist and elbow are in one line for extra support.

5. As you're lying in this position, notice where you're feeling this pose, and breathe slowly and deeply.

6. Inhale and on the exhale gently bring your right arm back into a tabletop position and then repeat on the other side.

7. You can alternate the arms and do four to five repetitions on each side. Try a few rounds with a couple of pauses when the arm is 'through the needle' and a few rounds without a pause as a flow of movements.

OPTIONAL THREAD THE NEEDLE

You can add to this pose by lifting your left arm into the air while your right arm is 'through the needle'. You can then bring your left arm over your head and place the palm of your left hand on the floor.

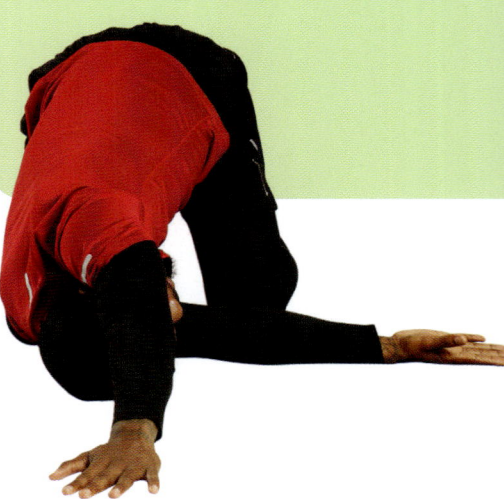

NOTE

You will feel this pose wherever there is tension in your body. However, as areas start to loosen up you will start noticing this in the space in between your spine and shoulder blade, on the side where your arm is down.

3   LOW LUNGE CACTUS ARMS

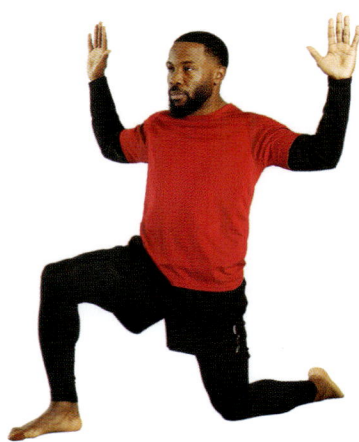
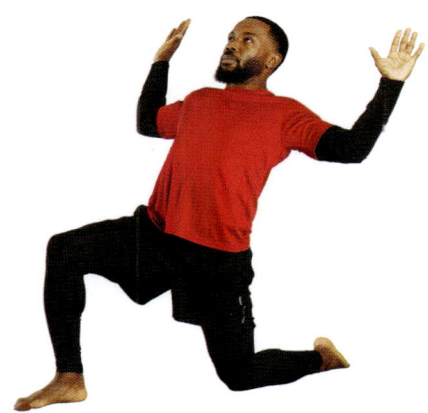

Low lunges are among my favourite poses. I suggest everyone performs them on a regular basis and you can do this pose several times a week – as you have probably noticed, variations on the low lunge have already appeared in these routines (see page 64).

The hip flexors and the lower back are directly interconnected through an arrangement of muscles and other soft tissue that join the pelvis and lower part of the spine together. Running, sprinting, changing direction and kicking the ball in particular can lead to an imbalance, reduced range of movement, tight hip flexors and subsequent lower back issues. By helping to lengthen the hip flexors, this pose improves flexibility and aids the release of tension in these muscles, all of which safeguard the hips and lower back.

1. Start in lunge position with your left knee and shin on the floor, and right leg forward with your foot on the mat and ankle and knee in one line.

2. Engage your core muscles by gently squeezing your belly button towards your spine. Keep your shoulders and hip stacked and in line, your spine long and your tail bone (the base of your spine) pointing down towards the floor, so your hips are in neutral and not tilting.

3. Inhale and as you exhale bring your arms out to the sides with your elbows bent and horizontally in line with your shoulders, and elbows and wrists in line vertically, with your palms facing forward.

4. Inhale and as you exhale lean slightly into your front leg to deepen the stretch in the hip flexors of your back leg, and/or very gently lean your chest and upper body back without arching your lower back too much. Notice how you're lengthening your hip flexors and the front of your body.

5. Hold this pose for two to three breaths or as long as it feels good.

6. Slowly release and repeat on the other side.

4 BRIDGE

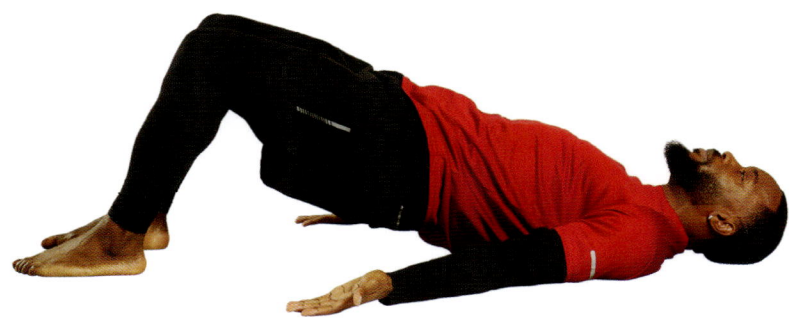

If you've ever had a lower body injury you probably know of the bridge as it is a very important exercise in any rehab or prehab programme. This pose improves spinal flexibility and opens up the front of the body in areas like the chest and the hips, while simultaneously strengthening the back of the body and the posterior chain – the muscles and connective tissues that run all the way from the back of the head down to the heels. Improving the strength, stability and flexibility of the posterior chain is key when we want to lower the risk of injuries, enhance performance and improve functional movement patterns.

1. Lie on your back with your legs bent at the knees and pointing up towards the ceiling, and feet on the floor. Your feet and knees should be hip-width apart, and your arms beside your body.

2. Inhale and on your exhale lift your hips up towards the ceiling while pressing into your feet and arms.

3. Keep your core and gluteus muscles engaged, and focus on slow and deep breaths.

4. You can stay with your arms on the floor or interlock your hands under your back and roll your shoulders to lift slightly higher into the bridge.

5. Hold the pose for 30 to 60 seconds.

6. Then very slowly lower your upper, middle and lower back down before allowing your hips to reach the floor.

7. Pause here and take a breath or two before repeating the pose.

8. Repeat for as many rounds as feel good.

07 LOWER BACK ROUTINE

NOTE
To make sure your knees don't move inwards or outwards during the pose you can keep a block between them.

As you move down and descend from the bridge, move so that your vertebrae come down one at a time. This supports spinal health since it allows the spine to release in a safe way and to gradually return to its natural curve, reducing the risk of compression or of force on the vertebrae or discs in between them.

MODIFIED BRIDGE

For an excellent restorative variation on this pose, place a bolster under your hips and hold the pose for three to five minutes. This helps decompress the spine and release tension in the lower back, enhancing flexibility in the hip joints and hip flexors. Additionally, focusing on deep, slow belly breaths calms the nervous system, reducing stress and promoting overall relaxation.

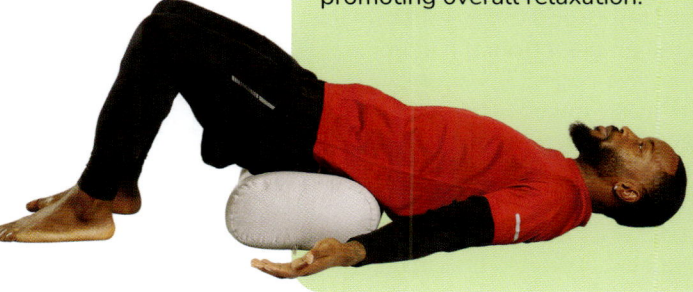

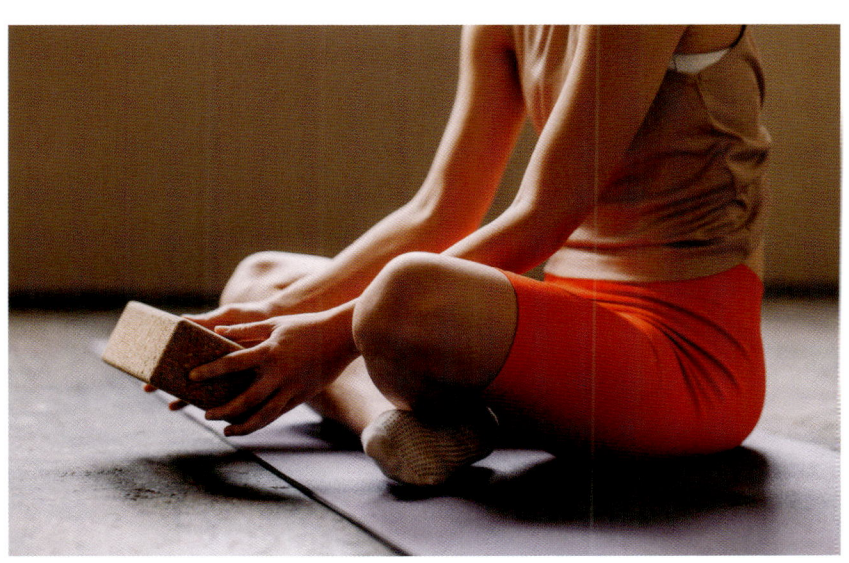

5 ROCK 'N' ROLLS

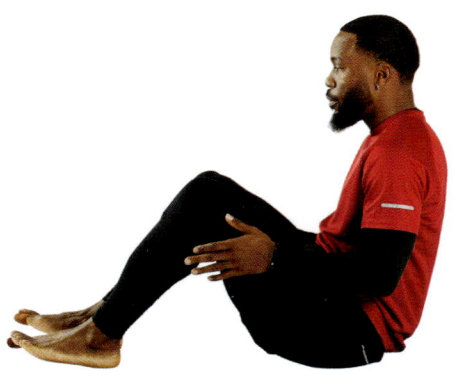
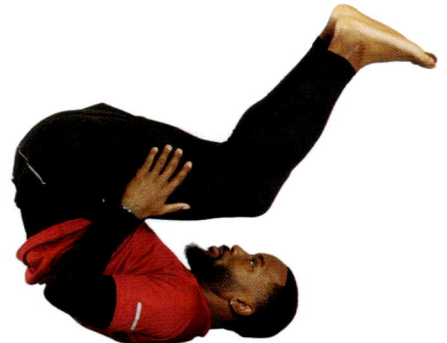

Rock 'n' rolls is another movement that is excellent to add to any routine – you may remember it from the morning routine (see page 33). I have included it here in the lower back routine since it really helps in releasing stiffness and tension in the spine, especially in the lower back area. The forward and backward rolling motion of the movement stimulates the circulation while gently massaging the spinal muscles, therefore improving the flexibility and mobility of the back.

1. Sit with your knees bent and your feet on the floor, keeping your hands gently on your legs, just below your knees.

2. Inhale and as you exhale rock backwards on to your back, lifting your feet and legs off the floor, and allowing your legs to move freely and as far or little back as feels natural.

3. On the same exhale, rock forwards by gently pressing your hands into your legs, and come on to your sit bones and initial position, keeping your spine nice and long.

4. Continue to rock backwards and forwards, allowing your breath to lead the movements, for as many times as it feels good.

07 LOWER BACK ROUTINE

6 LOCUST

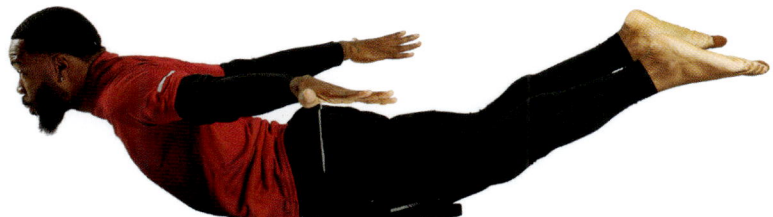

Just like the bridge, the locust is a great pose for strengthening the posterior chain – the calves, hamstrings, gluteus, and the spinal and back muscles. This pose also activates and engages the core and pelvis muscles, and when regularly practised it therefore helps players maintain a stable core and a strong centre of power, improve their spinal extension, and back strength and endurance, which all play a vital role in maintaining correct posture and hence preventing injuries during training sessions and games.

NOTE
You should not feel any pain in the lower back while in locust and if you do it's because you have lifted too much.

I also recommend rocking your hips gently from side to side in between each round. This releases any tension that has built up in the lower back during the pose, and encourages the soft tissue in the lumbar spine to relax and release any tightness. The rocking of the hips can also be added after any other pose when discomfort or tension in the lower back is felt.

1. Lie on your front with your legs extended, arms beside your body and palms facing down. Rest your forehead on the floor.

2. Inhale and as you exhale squeeze your core and belly button up towards your spine, lift your legs away from the floor and simultaneously lift your chest, arms and head.

3. Keep your eyes forward, but not too high up to avoid pain in the neck.

4. Hold this position for a few breaths, but make sure you keep your core engaged.

5. To release, slowly lower your arms and legs back to the floor.

6. Repeat for as many rounds as feels good, making sure that the core is engaged and activated throughout the full length of holding the pose.

7 REVERSED TABLETOP

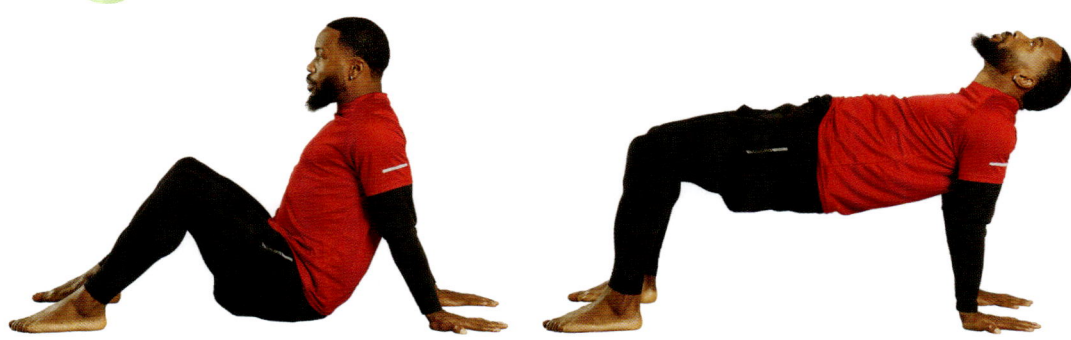

The reversed tabletop is an excellent pose for footballers since it strengthens and lengthens the major muscle groups involved in running, repeated changes of direction and kicking, while promoting the health of the lower back and spine.

Practise this regularly and you will benefit from an increase in your front-of-body muscles and lengthening in the chest, shoulders and hip flexor muscles, too. What's more, at the same time this will strengthen the muscles of the wrists, arms and core, and the back-of-the-body muscles, such as the glutes, hamstrings and lower back.

1. Sit in the middle of your mat with your feet flat on the floor and knees bent, hip-width apart.

2. Place your hands behind you on the mat and with your fingers pointing away from you, so from the side you look like a capital letter M.

3. Think about your core and hips taking off. Inhale and on your exhale press your hands and feet into the floor, and press yourself up and away from the mat as far as it feels comfortable.

4. Throughout the hold keep lifting your chest and hips, and feel the engagement of your core and gluteus muscles.

5. Hold the pose for a few breaths.

6. To release, slowly lower the hips back down to the floor, shake the wrists and arms out a little, and continue for another two to three rounds.

NOTE
If your shoulders are very tight it might initially not be possible to come into a full reversed tabletop. However, with regular practice, and as you become more flexible and supple, you will be able to go further into the pose.

8 COBRA PRESS-UPS

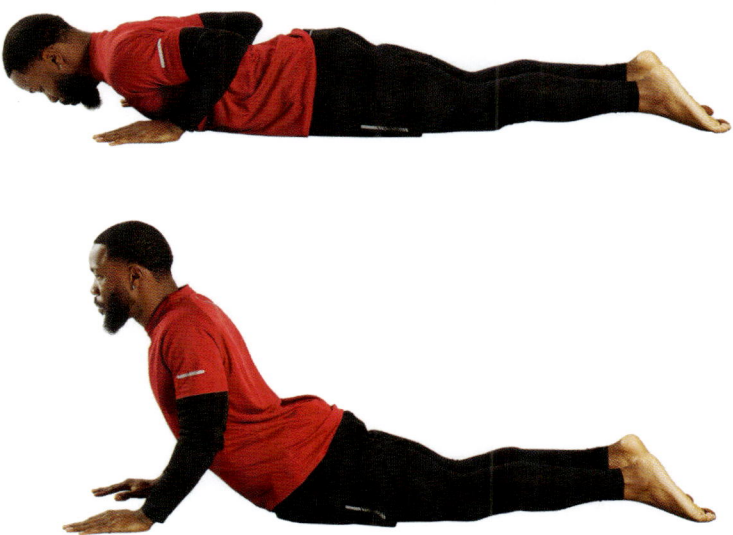

The cobra press-ups are another great movement to incorporate into your weekly training routine, especially if you have lower back issues. This exercise promotes spinal health by strengthening the surrounding muscles, and improving spinal flexibility and mobility, creating more space in the lower back. It helps counteract the repetitive movements that a footballer's body endures during intense training sessions or games, which often lead to muscle imbalances and result in tension or tightness in the lower back.

1. Lie on your front, with your legs extended, hands under your shoulders and elbows tucked into your body.

2. Inhale and as you exhale press into your hands and lift your chest, and your upper and middle abdominals, off the mat until your arms are almost straight, with a slight bend in the elbows.

3. In the same exhale, lower yourself back down.

4. Repeat this movement for eight to ten repetitions and for one to two sets, always breathing in when prone and exhaling as you move.

9 CHILD'S POSE TO COBRA FLOW

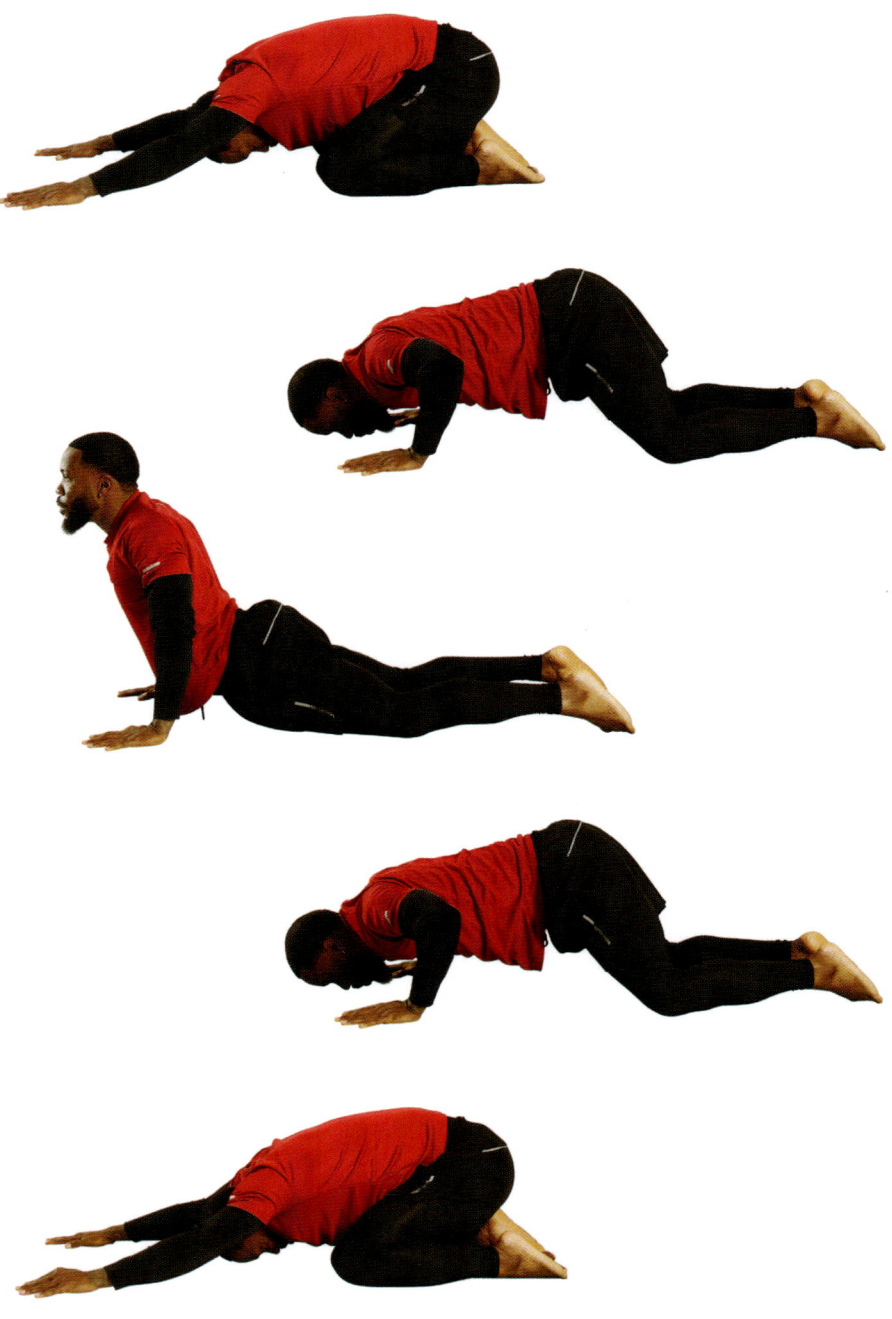

07 LOWER BACK ROUTINE

Due to the physical demands of football it is, as we all know, very common that the hips get tight and, as a result, for the shoulders and spine to become restricted. This is because the shoulders, hips and spine are interconnected through a network of muscles and other soft tissue, such as ligaments, tendons and fascia.

If one of those areas is tight or restricted it can create imbalances in other areas or even your entire body. It is therefore important that it all functions as connected parts and works well together, so your body can support your posture, stability and movement, and ultimately help you to prevent injuries and maintain your optimal performance.

This child's pose to cobra sequence is included in this lower back routine because it targets the shoulders, hips and spine, and addresses the interconnection of these areas, improving mobility while simultaneously providing a complete lengthening and release of tension in all those areas, and hence restoring balance in the body. As with any flowing movement it also encourages conscious breathing and mindfulness, nurturing a stronger connection between the body and mind.

1. Sit in child's pose (see page 80) with your shins on the floor, knees bent and wider than hip-width apart, hips moved back towards your heels, big toes touching and arms in front of you on the mat, palms down.

2. Inhale and on your exhale slowly move forwards on to the mat, with your chest and face close to the floor, as if your nose is leading the movement and almost touching the mat as you come into prone position with your palms right under your shoulders.

3. Inhale and on the exhale press your palms into the mat and lift your upper body off the floor, straightening your arms, and keeping your elbows tucked in to your body.

4. Inhale and lower your upper body back down to the floor.

5. Engage your core and, as you exhale, lift your hips up and move back into child's pose. On your way, keep your chest and face close to the floor.

6. Repeat this for five to ten rounds. Allow a smooth flow between child's pose and cobra. You can do the flow slower or faster, or allow the rhythm of your breath to be the rhythm of your movement, but try to find smoothness in your movement.

7. Once you have finished the rounds, stay in child's pose for a couple of minutes. Breathe deeply and relax.

08 CORE ROUTINE

1. Dead bug movement .... page 134
2. Rock 'n' rolls .... page 135
3. Bird dog .... page 136
4. Boat .... page 137
5. Single arm/leg plank .... page 138
6. Yoga side plank .... page 140
7. One-legged dog flow ...... page 142
8. Dolphin .... page 144
9. Warrior 2 .... page 145

A combination of traditional exercises and yoga can challenge your core to stabilise your body – this is key to dynamic on-pitch movement.

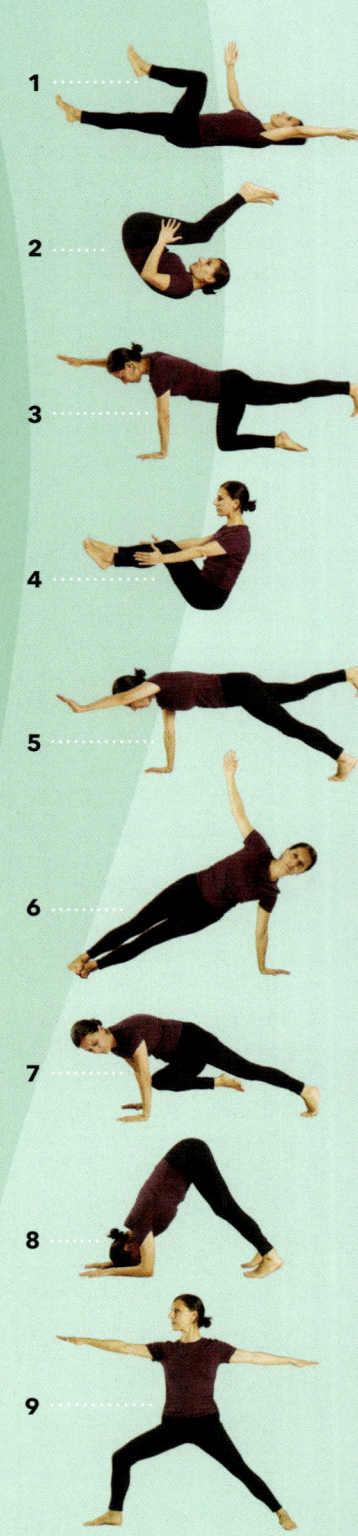

08 CORE ROUTINE

Having a strong core is vital when playing football. This is the centre of your power and it is from here that you generate the energy needed to maintain high levels of performance. A strong core allows you to control your movements on the pitch efficiently, transfer power between your upper and lower body, and maintain good balance.

Integrating yoga poses into a conventional exercise programme helps to develop core stability and strength, while also improving your body's coordination. These poses not only engage the deeper core muscles, but also promote balance and endurance, which are crucial during high-intensity gameplay.

This holistic approach to core training supports a strong, stable spine and can aid in easing or preventing lower back pain. Incorporating these postures into your routine not only enhances your core strength, but also improves flexibility, balance and muscular endurance, all of which contribute to more powerful, controlled and injury-resistant performances on the pitch.

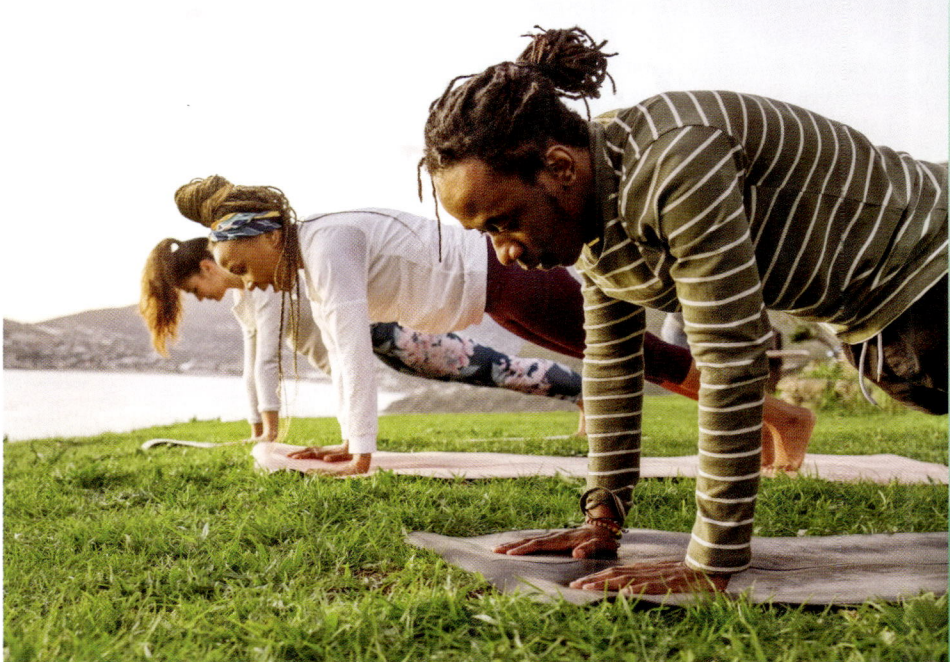

1 DEAD BUG MOVEMENT

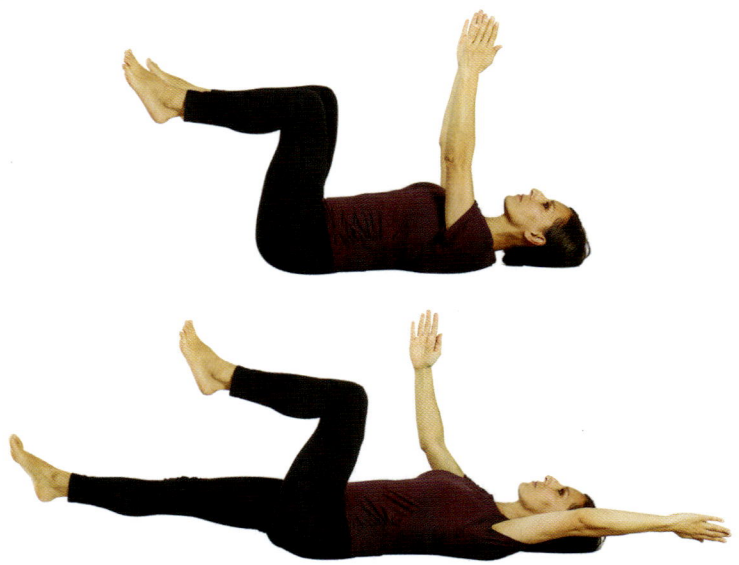

The dead bug is great for footballers as it is an extremely effective core stability and strengthening exercise. It is especially beneficial for those needing to develop their core strength and endurance, improve their posture and alignment, reduce the risk of injuries, and come back from hip and spinal injuries. The dead bug movement is highly recommended and a great tool to add to any rehab, prehab or conditioning programme.

1. Lie on your back with your knees bent at 90 degrees, the front of your thighs facing you and the lower part of your legs parallel to the floor, with your arms straight up towards the ceiling, your wrist, elbows and shoulders in a line.

2. Gently squeeze your belly button down towards your spine and the floor to engage your core. It is very important that your core is engaged throughout this whole movement, so keep your lower back gently pressed into the floor the whole time.

3. Inhale and on the exhale squeeze your core and then slowly extend and lower your right leg towards the floor, at the same time as you extend and lower your left arm down.

4. Inhale and on your exhale come back to the middle point with your arm and leg.

5. Repeat on the other side, always starting with an inhale and squeezing the core on the exhale, before moving the limbs.

6. As with everything, quality is much more important than quantity here. Start with two sets of six to eight repetitions on each side and then increase as you feel your core getting stronger.

2 ROCK 'N' ROLLS

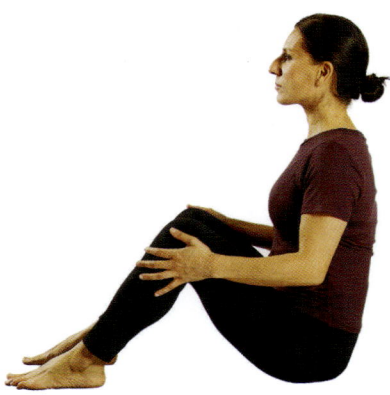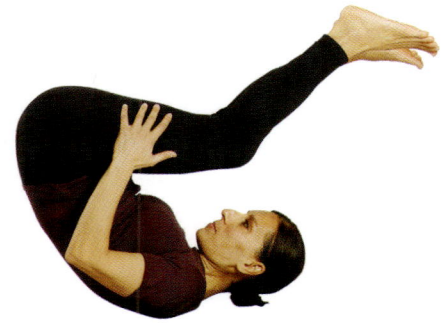

An excellent movement to incorporate into your core routine, rock 'n' rolls can be practised at any time of the day. It not only engages your core, but also helps release stiffness and tension in the spine, particularly in the lower back. The forward and backward rolling action stimulates circulation, gently massages the spinal muscles, and enhances flexibility and mobility. It's a great way to warm up the core and spine before more intense exercises or to cool down and relieve tension after a demanding session.

1. Sit with your knees bent and your feet on the floor, keeping your hands gently on your legs, just below your knees.

2. Inhale and as you exhale rock backwards on to your back, lifting your feet and legs off the floor, and allowing your legs to move freely and as far or little back as feels natural.

3. On the same exhale, rock forwards by gently pressing your hands into your legs, and come on to your sit bones and initial position, keeping your spine nice and long.

4. Continue to rock backwards and forwards, allowing your breath to lead the movements, for as many times as it feels good.

3 BIRD DOG

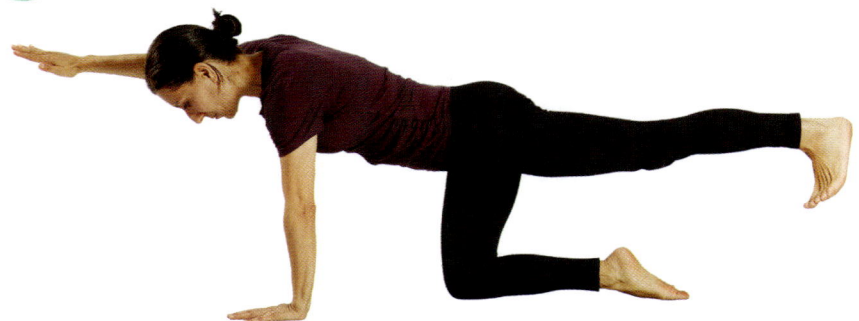

The bird dog is simple yet versatile and effective, but although the movement looks easy to perform, it requires stability and focus to execute it correctly. It targets the core, lower back and gluteus muscles, at the same time as enhancing your proprioception – balance and coordination. You might know it if you have previously been injured, since it is usually included in rehab programmes, but it makes a good addition to any weekly routine.

1. Begin on your hands and knees, in a tabletop position. Make sure your wrists, elbows and shoulders are in line, and your knees are below your hips, hip-width apart.

2. Inhale and on your exhale extend your right arm forward and your left leg back, keeping them in line with each other and your body.

3. Keep your hips squared and core engaged by gently pulling your belly button up towards your spine. Imagine a glass of water on your lower back and try to keep it there the entire time without spilling it.

4. Hold this pose for a couple of breaths.

5. Release and come back to your tabletop position. Inhale and on the exhale repeat on the other side. Do four to eight rounds.

08 CORE ROUTINE

4 BOAT

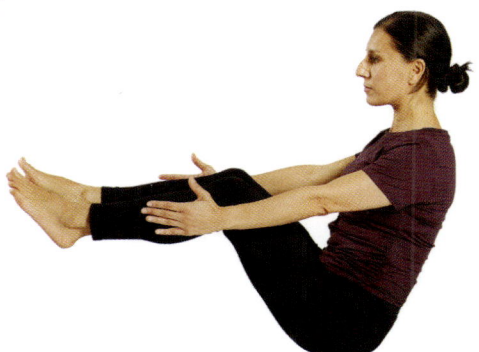

Boat is an excellent posture that not only strengthens the entire core, but also activates the spine, hip flexors and lower leg muscles. This makes it particularly beneficial for increasing speed and overall endurance. Holding the pose, especially with the legs straight, can be challenging and demands a combination of strength, coordination and balance, as it engages different muscle groups simultaneously.

1. Sit on your mat with your knees bent, your feet on the floor and your hands resting on the mat beside your hips.

2. Keeping your spine straight, lean back slightly and lift your feet off the mat.

3. Inhale and on the exhale extend and straighten your legs, creating a letter V shape with your body. If this is too intense, you can keep your knees bent like in the above picture.

4. Keep your core engaged by gently pulling your belly button towards your spine, your chest lifted and your eyes looking forward.

5. Extend your arms in front of you, shoulders to wrists in one line, and palms facing each other.

6. Stay here for 15 to 30 seconds, focusing on slow and deep breaths.

7. Slowly release by bringing your feet back down and repeat if you want to.

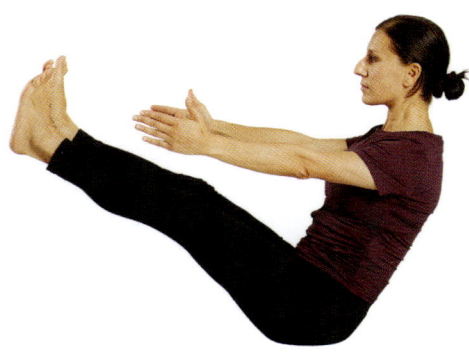

NOTE

If you're new to this pose or coming back from injury in the core or surrounding areas, it is advisable to initially start by staying in the opening phase with knees bent and feet off the floor. Once your core is feeling stronger you can 'play' with the pose and start bending or extending one leg out at a time, before going into the full pose.

5 SINGLE ARM/LEG PLANK

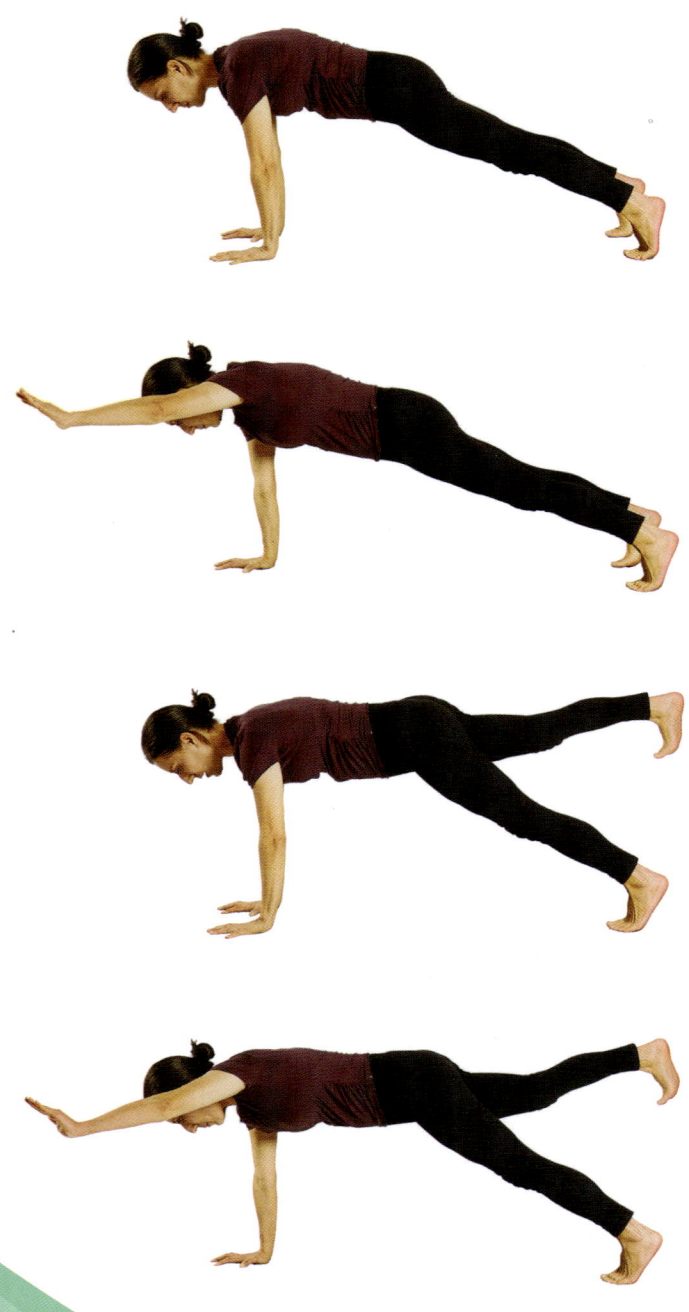

08 CORE ROUTINE

The single arm/leg plank is particularly effective as it not only strengthens the deep stabilising muscles crucial for dynamic movements on the pitch, but also simultaneously engages both the upper and lower body muscles.

This excellent variation of the plank enhances overall stability and balance. Like the traditional yoga plank (see page 44), it is beneficial for footballers as it works a broad range of muscle groups, including the core, glutes, upper back, chest, shoulders, arms and wrists, while promoting healthier spinal and pelvic alignment. Both variations improve stability and control, especially in the shoulders and hips, which are essential for maintaining power and balance during dynamic movements.

1. Begin on your hands and knees, in a tabletop position. Make sure your wrists, elbows and shoulders are in line, and your knees are below your hips, hip-width apart.

2. Inhale and on the exhale bring your legs back, one at a time, keeping them straight, with your heels above and in line with the base of your toes.

3. Activate your core muscles – imagine you're lifting your belly button up and in towards the spine.

4. Gently shift your weight forward, allowing your shoulders to be slightly over your wrists.

5. Keep your neck and head in line with your spine, and your gaze soft, looking slightly in front of you.

6. Shift your weight on to your right hand and, while keeping your spine and hips in line and your core strong to maintain stability, lift your left arm away from the floor and extend it in front of you.

7. Hold this position for a breath or two, while focusing on deep and slow breaths.

8. Slowly bring your arm back down to the floor, checking everything is in line again, and repeat with the right arm. Hold for the same number of breaths.

9. Then do the same with the legs, one leg at a time. Both hands should be down.

10. To progress, you can lift an opposite arm and leg simultaneously, and then repeat with the other arm and leg.

NOTE
In your plank, think about keeping your body in a straight line, from your head all the way to your heels, and focus on your breath.

YOGA FOR FOOTBALLERS

6 YOGA SIDE PLANK

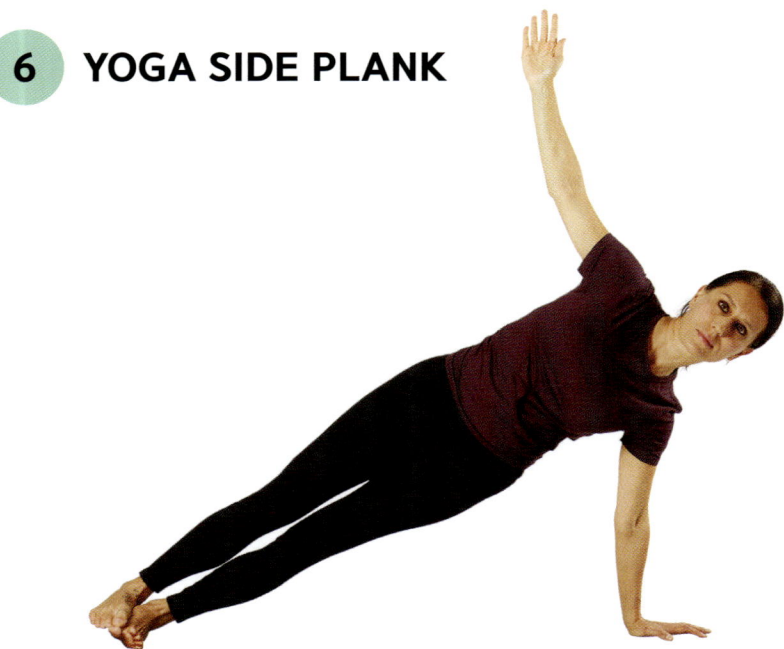

The yoga side plank is a valuable addition to a core routine for footballers and can help prepare you for the physical demands of the game and enhance your overall performance. This challenging pose enhances functional strength, stability and balance – essential components for optimal performance on the pitch. By improving agility, power and injury resilience, the side plank helps players maintain balance and control during dynamic situations, such as holding off an opponent with an extended arm.

1. Start in a yoga plank (see page 44), keeping a straight line from the top of your head to your heels, with your wrists, elbows and shoulders aligned.

2. Move your weight on to your left hand and the edge of your left foot. From here, you can either stack your right foot on top of the left one or place it on the floor slightly in front of the left, which will give you more stability.

3. Inhale and as you exhale gently lift yourself up, making sure your hips are lifted and in line with your shoulder and your left wrist, elbow and shoulder are aligned.

4. Move your right arm up towards the ceiling so that it forms a straight line with your shoulders.

5. Hold this pose for 15 to 30 seconds, or longer if it feels comfortable and you're in good alignment.

6. Focus on your breath, breathing deeply and slowly, in and out.

7. When you're ready to release, bring your right arm back down on to the floor, so you come into a plank. Then switch on to your right arm and repeat on the other side.

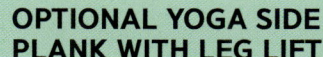

OPTIONAL YOGA SIDE PLANK WITH LEG LIFT

When performing the yoga side plank with your top leg lifted, you further enhance and deepen your core stability. This variation also strengthens the hip abductors, improving balance and resistance against lateral forces, which are crucial for efficient lateral movements and stability on the pitch. To perform it, do the initial steps of the side plank and then, once you have found stability, inhale and on the exhale lift your left leg up and away from the right one, keeping your hips square and core engaged. Focus on a point in front of you, which will help with your balance, and hold the pose for a few breaths. Slowly lower your top leg, return to the plank pose and repeat on the other side.

MODIFIED YOGA SIDE PLANK WITH LEG LIFT

A great variation for beginners or those who are coming back from an injury and have restricted mobility and/or strength, this modified yoga side plank is performed just like the side plank, with the right hand on the floor and the right arm straight, with the left arm straight and up in the air, and the shoulders stacked. The difference, though, is that the right knee is bent and rests on the ground, which keeps the pelvis and hips more stable. Once you feel stable in the pose lift your top leg away from the floor and in the air, so the top foot, knee and hips are in one line.

7 ONE-LEGGED DOG FLOW

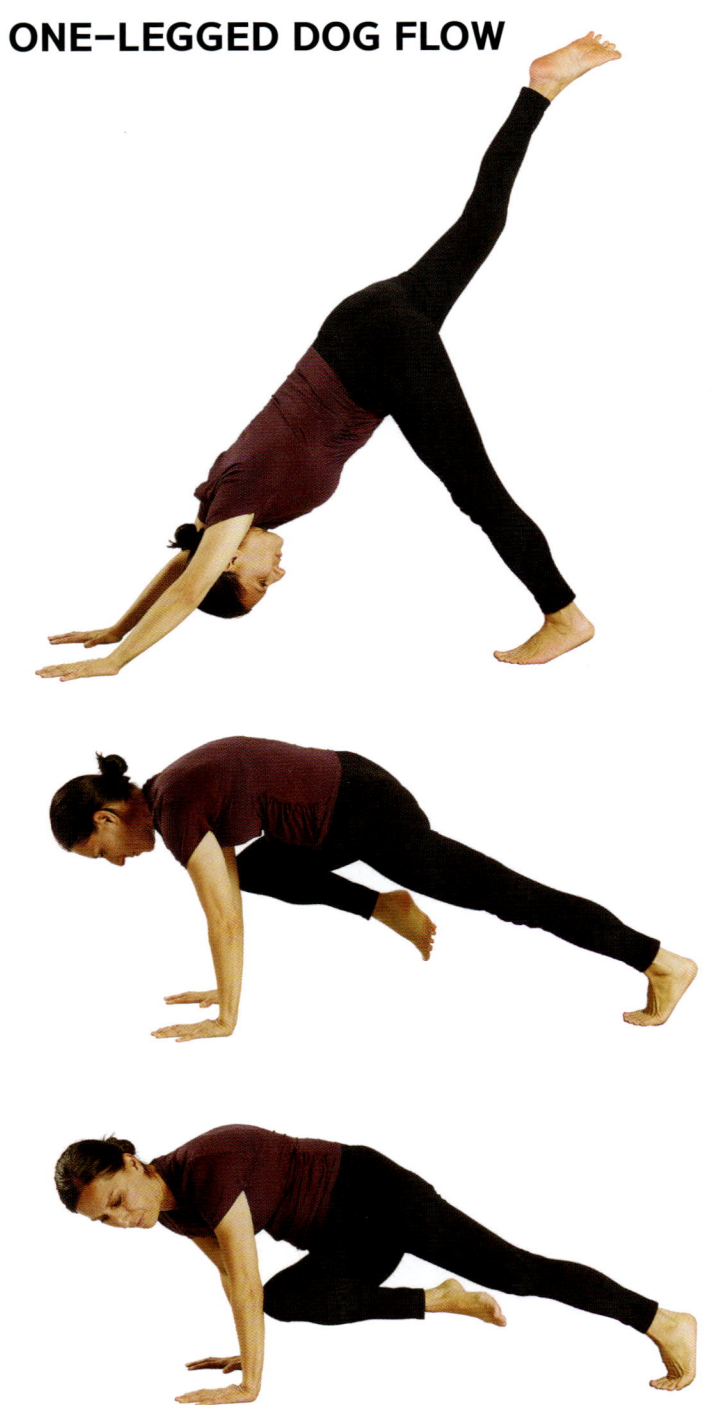

08 CORE ROUTINE

This dynamic flow is an excellent combination for core stability and strengthening. The sequence improves balance and coordination while building functional strength and endurance throughout the entire body by engaging multiple muscle groups. Additionally, it lengthens the back of the body, making it a comprehensive and effective workout. This makes it highly beneficial and I recommend everyone includes it in their core programmes.

1. Start in downward-facing dog (see page 48) with your hips high up, knees slightly bent, feet hip-width apart and hands shoulder-width apart.

2. Inhale and on your exhale bring your right leg straight up towards the ceiling, keeping your hips square.

3. Hold this position – one-legged dog – for a breath and notice the right glute being engaged.

4. Inhale and as you exhale bring your weight forward as if you're coming into a one-legged yoga plank, at the same time moving your right knee to touch your right elbow.

5. Hold for a breath and notice how your whole body, core and obliques are working.

6. On an exhale bring your leg back up in the air. Inhale and exhale forward into a one-legged yoga plank, this time moving your right knee to touch your left elbow. Pause for a breath.

7. Slowly bring your right leg back up, before moving it back down and returning to a downward-facing dog.

8. Repeat on the other side and do one to five rounds or as many as feels good.

NOTE
To progress or make the pose more challenging, touch your knee slightly above your elbows and/or pause for longer.

8 DOLPHIN

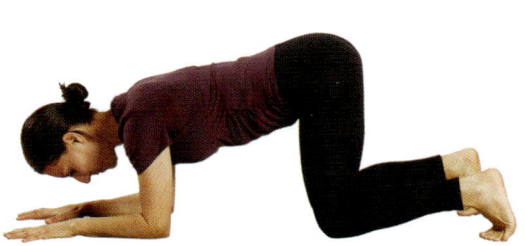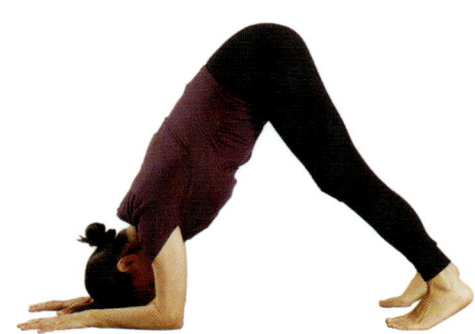

The dolphin resembles downward-facing dog, but is performed on the forearms, which allows it to engage and strengthen the core muscles even more effectively. It also enhances stability and strength in the upper body, shoulders and back.

Like downward-facing dog, dolphin provides flexibility benefits by lengthening and reducing tension in the glutes, hamstrings and calf muscles. This, in turn, encourages improved spinal alignment and supports spinal health.

NOTE
Ideally you need to keep your knees straight in this pose, but if your upper back rounds it's better to keep your knees slightly bent.

Sometimes it's also hard to keep your arms parallel to each other throughout. If that is the case, you can interlock your hands while still keeping your elbows in line with and underneath the shoulders.

It is always good to finish the dolphin pose with a child's pose (see page 80), held for a few slow breaths.

1. Begin on your hands and knees, in a tabletop position. Make sure your wrists, elbows and shoulders are in line, and your knees are below your hips, hip-width apart.

2. Inhale and on your exhale lower your forearms to the floor, parallel to each other.

3. Inhale and tuck your toes in, exhale and lift your hips up high. Start walking your feet a little closer towards your arms, so your hips reach even higher up towards the ceiling and your legs are even straighter.

4. Keep your forearms active by pressing them into the floor.

5. Allow your head to rest between your arms and keep your eyes towards your feet.

6. Hold the pose for 15 to 30 seconds or longer, while focusing on deep and slow breaths.

7. To release, slowly lower your knees to the floor and repeat if you want.

9 WARRIOR 2

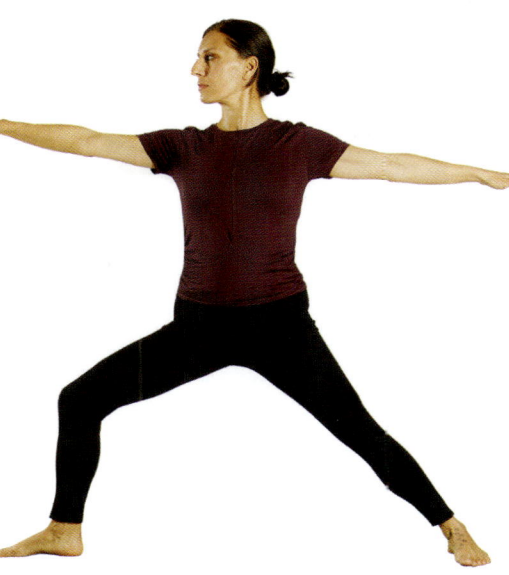

You have already met warrior 1 (see page 96) and warrior 3 (see page 53). Warrior 2 is an equally powerful pose and it appears in this routine because it not only activates your core but also focuses on pelvic stability and alignment, while simultaneously strengthening everything above and below. These elements are crucial in any core programme since everything in the body is interconnected.

In warrior 2 you benefit from strengthening the leg muscles – the quadriceps, hamstrings and glutes – while also engaging and strengthening the hip muscles and improving hip mobility. Improved strength and flexibility in these areas can enhance performance, improve stability during movements and reduce the risk of injury.

Performing this pose correctly requires full concentration, so practising it regularly can improve focus during a game, leading to better awareness and decision-making on the pitch. Adding it to your practice has the potential to enhance your overall performance, resulting in excellent endurance, agility and coordination during training sessions or games.

1. Stand at the front of your mat. Inhale and on your exhale step your left leg back about a metre. Keep the toes of your right foot pointing forwards and your left foot turned, with those toes pointing to the long side of the mat.

2. Inhale and as you exhale bend your right knee, making sure your knee and ankle are in one line. You might need to bring your left leg slightly further away to line up the front knee and ankle. Check that the middle of your front knee is in line with your second and third toe, so your knee is not moving inwards.

3. Bring your arms up and extend them to the sides, keeping them parallel to the floor and palms facing down.

4. Look towards your front fingertips. Imagine you're a warrior standing strong with your arms moving away from each other, core and trunk engaged, leg muscles both strengthening and lengthening.

5. Focus on breathing slowly and deeply, while holding the pose for a few breaths.

6. To release, inhale and on your exhale come back to the front of the mat. Pause for a breath then repeat on the other side.

09 RELAXATION ROUTINE

1. Diaphragmatic breath ...... page 148
2. Alternate nostril breathing .... page 149
3. Bee breath .... page 150
4. Twisting crouching tiger ... page 151
5. Supported fish .... page 152
6. Bananasana .... page 153

Proper relaxation is essential to transform potential into peak performance, whether on or off the pitch.

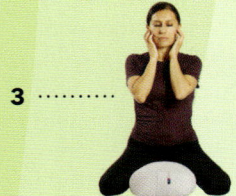

1

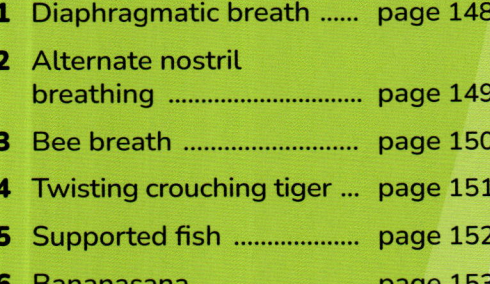

2

3

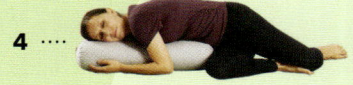

4

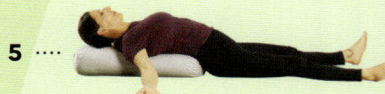

5

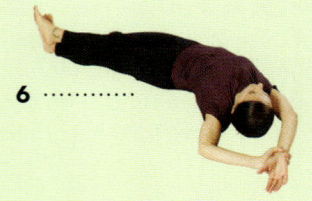

6

09 RELAXATION ROUTINE

Like the evening routine, this relaxation routine is calming and restorative, but it offers you different options and is a great addition to your training schedule if, for example, you're going through a challenging period, on or off the pitch, or your body and mind need a more soothing practice.

This routine gives you three different breathwork techniques. These will improve respiratory muscle strength and efficiency, which supports better oxygen uptake, removal of carbon dioxide, and overall wellbeing and function of the respiratory system. These functions are essential for athletic performance – delivering sufficient oxygen to working muscles during training or a game enhances your aerobic capacity, endurance and stamina, allowing you to withstand high-intensity exertions for longer periods of time.

Breathwork also helps regulate your heart rate and activate the parasympathetic nervous system, which governs digestion and rest. Once the body and mind are relaxed, the digestive organs can absorb nutrients, stress levels lower, and mental and physical recovery is enhanced.

Explore how you can integrate these breathwork techniques into your daily routines, not just your relaxation routine – as part of your pre-training/pre-match routine, for example, they can help you increase focus, concentration and emotional regulation.

Alongside breathwork, restorative yoga is a gentle practice that focuses on deep relaxation and the release of tension in both the body and mind. During restorative postures, equipment like bolsters, bricks and blankets are used for support and comfort, and the poses are held for extended periods. This approach enhances the circulation and elasticity of connective tissue and fascia, promoting flexibility and lengthening. As a result, players experience improved range of motion and a decreased risk of injury.

Furthermore, restorative postures are profoundly calming and offer much more than mere rest. They provide an opportunity for you to relax, breathe slowly and be fully present in the moment. They are deeply soothing and allow your body to enter a state of calmness. When this happens, your muscles release tension and your breath slows down. As tension is released and breathing becomes deeper and slower, your mind begins to relax. At this point, your body starts releasing serotonin and dopamine – the feel-good hormones. Suddenly, life feels lighter.

YOGA FOR FOOTBALLERS

DIAPHRAGMATIC BREATH

This breathing technique is a simple yet effective way of promoting relaxation and can be performed literally anywhere and at any time. By pausing for a moment in the course of your day and taking 10 to 20 diaphragmatic breaths, you will activate your parasympathetic nervous system, encouraging relaxation and stress reduction, and giving your mind a moment to ground and centre, for example during an intense game, when it is vital to maintain your concentration. It also improves oxygen exchange, allowing the lungs to better take in oxygen, while driving out carbon dioxide, which in turn boosts the efficiency of the lungs.

By including this breathwork in your daily routine and creating short spells of relaxation while optimising your oxygen uptake, you can also help your body to recover faster when off the pitch, and enhance your stamina and performance on the pitch.

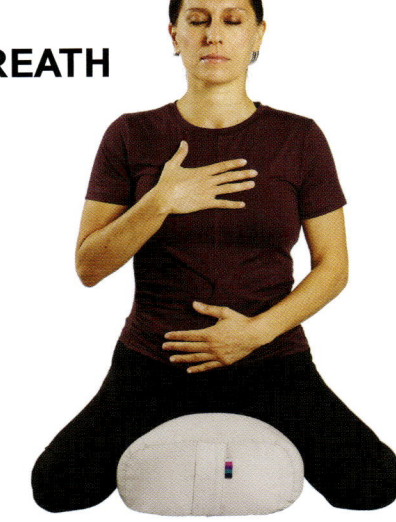

1. Find a comfortable position, either sitting or lying down.

2. Place one hand on your chest and the other on your lower belly.

3. Breathe deeply in through your nose, or mouth, and all the way down to your belly, feeling how your abdomen rises into your hand while the hand on your chest is somewhat still.

4. Slowly breathe out through your mouth and feel how your belly goes back down and empties under your hand.

5. Repeat this breath 10 to 20 times, or for longer if it feels good.

AVOID IF...

You have a heart condition; a severe back or rib injury; you have recently undergone a hernia surgery; or you're pregnant (especially in the third trimester). If you have any of these conditions or any health concerns, speak to your doctor or health care provider before doing diaphragmatic breath or any of the breath techniques in this book.

NOTE

If you're totally new to this breath it might take a while for you to be able to breathe into your belly and you might feel your chest rises instead. This is normal and will change as you continue to practise, and pay full attention to your breath. Think about breathing slowly and deeply. The length of your inhale or exhale can be the same or your exhale can be longer. Find what feels good for you.

2 ALTERNATE NOSTRIL BREATHING

I recommend you perform this simple yet powerful breathwork before a game, particularly a big game, since it is a great tool for decreasing anxiety, while promoting calmness, and enhancing concentration and mental clarity. This technique is also fantastic when performed at half time, to mentally recharge you before you run back on to the pitch, or post-game to help you relax and recover more efficiently, physically and mentally.

To continue enjoying the remarkable benefits of this breathwork – such as improved mental clarity, stress reduction, overall respiratory health, enhanced physical and mental performance, and balanced brain hemispheres for better cognitive function – I suggest incorporating this excellent practice into your daily routine.

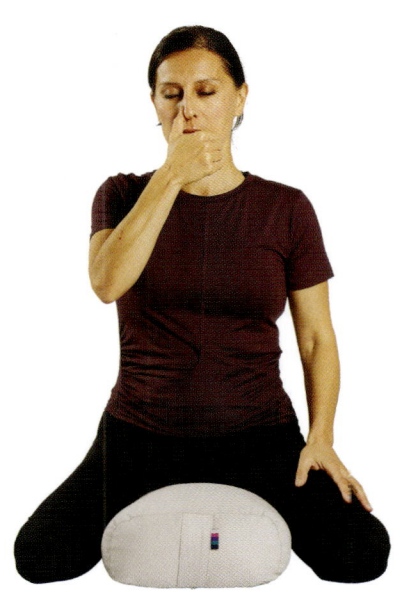

1. Find a comfortable place to sit. Keep your spine upright, and shoulders and face relaxed, with space between your jaws.

2. Take a couple of deep breaths in through your nose and out through your mouth, then keep your mouth closed for the rest of the exercise.

3. Using your right hand, close your right nostril with your thumb, breathing deeply and gently in through your left nostril.

4. Using your right index finger, close your left nostril, release your right nostril and fully exhale.

5. Keep your left nostril closed and breathe in through your right nostril.

AVOID IF...

You have high blood pressure; heart conditions; you suffer with severe headaches or migraines; you have had recent surgery or injury to your neck, head or nasal area; or you're pregnant (especially in the third trimester) and new to this technique. If you have any of these conditions or any health concerns, speak to your doctor or health care provider before doing alternate nostril breathing or any of the breath techniques in this book.

6. Close your right nostril, release your left nostril and fully exhale. This is one round.

7. Repeat this cycle for five to eight rounds, or more or fewer if that suits you better.

3 BEE BREATH

This is another amazing breathing technique that can be performed before games or at half time. Bee breath is an excellent tool that only takes a moment – it is probably the quickest breathing technique of them all – but it is very strong and potent, and delivers quick relaxation during moments of elevated stress.

The humming sound has a calming effect on the nervous system, which helps reduce stress and releases tension in the body and mind. This overall calmness boosts mental clarity, aids concentration and enhances decision-making.

1. Find a comfortable place to sit. Keep your spine upright, and your shoulders and face relaxed, with space between your jaws.

2. Take a couple of deep breaths in through your nose and out through your mouth, then keep your mouth closed for the rest of the exercise.

3. Close your eyes and place your index fingers over each ear, gently closing them in.

4. Inhale deeply through your nose.

5. Exhale through your nose while making a humming sound like a bee, generating a soft and consistent vibration that you can feel in your body and face. The humming sound should be smooth, steady and continuous, and you should exhale fully until you feel there is no air left to hum out.

6. Repeat this for six breaths.

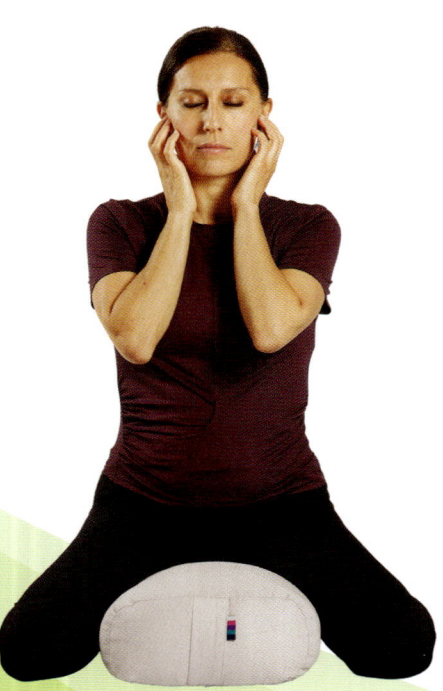

AVOID IF...

You have heart conditions; you suffer with severe headaches or migraines; you have had recent surgery to your abdomen, chest, neck or head; or you're pregnant (especially in the third trimester) and new to breathwork. If you have any of these conditions or any health concerns, speak to your doctor or health care provider before doing the bee breath or any of the breath techniques in this book.

4 TWISTING CROUCHING TIGER

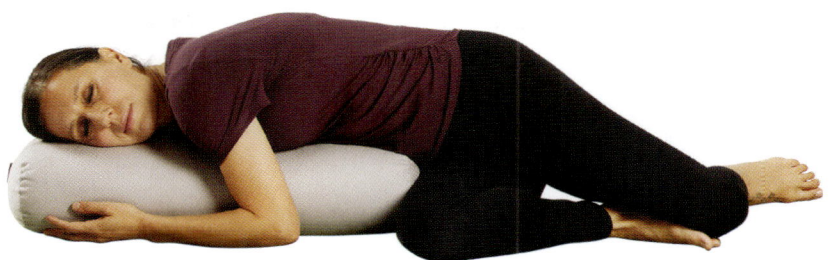

This is a favourite restorative pose. It gently allows the spine to twist, and creates space in the spinal and surrounding areas, supporting any discomfort in those areas, including the lower back, improving mobility, flexibility, alignment and spinal health. This pose is held for a longer time and this restorative aspect is meditative, and helps nurture mindfulness, which promotes relaxation. A regular practice calms the nervous system and helps to reduce stress and anxiety, so, for example, it's a great pose to perform after a high-pressure game.

1. Place a bolster or sturdy pillow vertically on your mat. Sit with your right outer hip next to the bottom part of the bolster, with your knees bent to the left.

2. Inhale and as you exhale twist your torso towards the bolster, so you're facing it.

3. Keep your hands on the floor either side of the bolster and slowly lower your upper body down on to it. Keep your arms wherever they feel comfortable.

4. Rest your right cheek on the bolster, so you're facing the same direction as your knees. Allow your body to fully relax into the pose.

5. Focus on slow and deep breaths, allowing any tension to release with each exhale.

6. Hold the pose for three to five minutes.

7. To release, slowly press the floor with your hands to come up. Take a moment and then repeat on the other side.

NOTE
Once you're used to this pose, and if you like more intensity, you can face the opposite direction to your knees.

5 SUPPORTED FISH

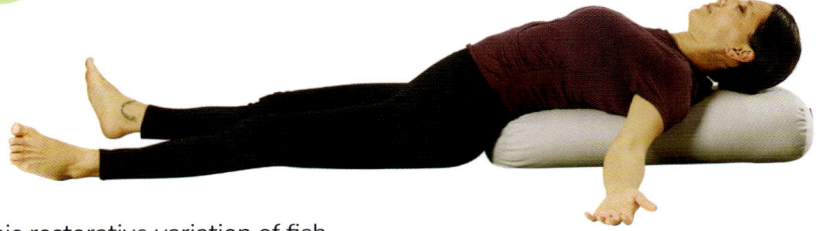

This restorative variation of fish pose is an excellent choice for rest and relaxation. Footballers often experience tightness in the chest and shoulder areas, not only due to the high demands of football training, but also from spending hours in the gym, with many players focusing too much on heavy upper body workouts.

Additionally, the long hours we all spend in seated positions – whether in cars, on coaches, trains, sofas or while using mobile phones – leads to a forward-hunched posture. This posture causes the shoulders to curl inward and tightens the chest and hip flexors. Unfortunately, there is often little or no time spent on exercises to counteract these effects and maintain openness and flexibility in these areas.

NOTE
Depending on the size of your bolster and the tension in the front of your body, your arms might not touch the floor. If that is the case, place a pillow or blanket on either side of you, so that your arms can reach down and rest.

Again, depending on the size of your bolster, you might feel that there is a lot of space between the lower part of your spine or the back of your hips and the floor, so you might be more comfortable if you place a small pillow or blanket under that area.

This is precisely what supported fish accomplishes: it opens the chest and shoulders, gently stretches the hip flexors, and improves posture, range of motion and breathing. This pose opens the front line of the body and relieves tightness in key areas, making it a valuable tool for supporting the physical and mental demands of both football and everyday life.

1. Sit in the middle of your mat with your legs stretched out in front of you. Place a bolster vertically behind you.

2. Inhale and as you exhale rest on to your bolster, allowing the back of your head, neck, and upper, middle and lower back to settle on the midline of the bolster.

3. Stretch your arms out to the side and allow your elbows to rest on the floor.

4. Gently close your eyes and focus on deep and slow breaths, noticing how the tension in the front of your body is releasing with each exhale.

5. Stay in this position for three to five minutes.

6. To come out of the pose, hug your arms in for a moment before gently rolling over to one side and slowly sitting up.

09 RELAXATION ROUTINE

6 BANANASANA

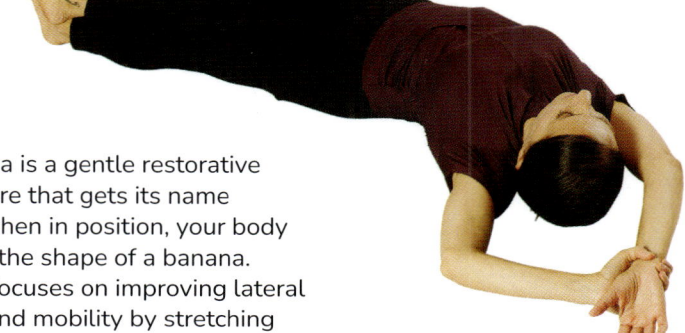

Bananasana is a gentle restorative yoga posture that gets its name because, when in position, your body resembles the shape of a banana. This pose focuses on improving lateral flexibility and mobility by stretching and creating space in the side body, including the outer hips, obliques, ribs and shoulders, while promoting relaxation.

By opening the ribcage, bananasana enhances breathing efficiency and supports better posture, both of which are fundamental for maintaining stamina and focus during the later stages of matches. The enhancement of lateral flexibility and mobility leads to improved movement on the pitch, increasing agility and allowing players to change direction more effectively and quickly during a game.

Thanks to its calming nature, this pose effectively reduces stress and encourages mental clarity as well, equipping players with the focus and composure needed during intense times. This combination of physical and mental benefits makes bananasana an invaluable addition to footballers' routines.

1. Lie flat on your back, with your arms beside your body and legs straight.

2. As you exhale, slide your legs to the left. To deepen the stretch, you can cross your right ankle over your left one.

3. Inhale and on your exhale reach your arms overhead, keeping them on the floor. Move them to your left, holding opposite wrists, and making sure your shoulders are relaxed, down and away from your ears.

4. Hold this position for three to five minutes, and breathe slowly and deeply. Relax into the pose and feel how the right side of your body is gently opening up with each exhale.

5. To release, slowly let go of your wrists and gently return your legs to the middle. Take a moment and then repeat on the other side.

SLEEP FOR PEAK PERFORMANCE

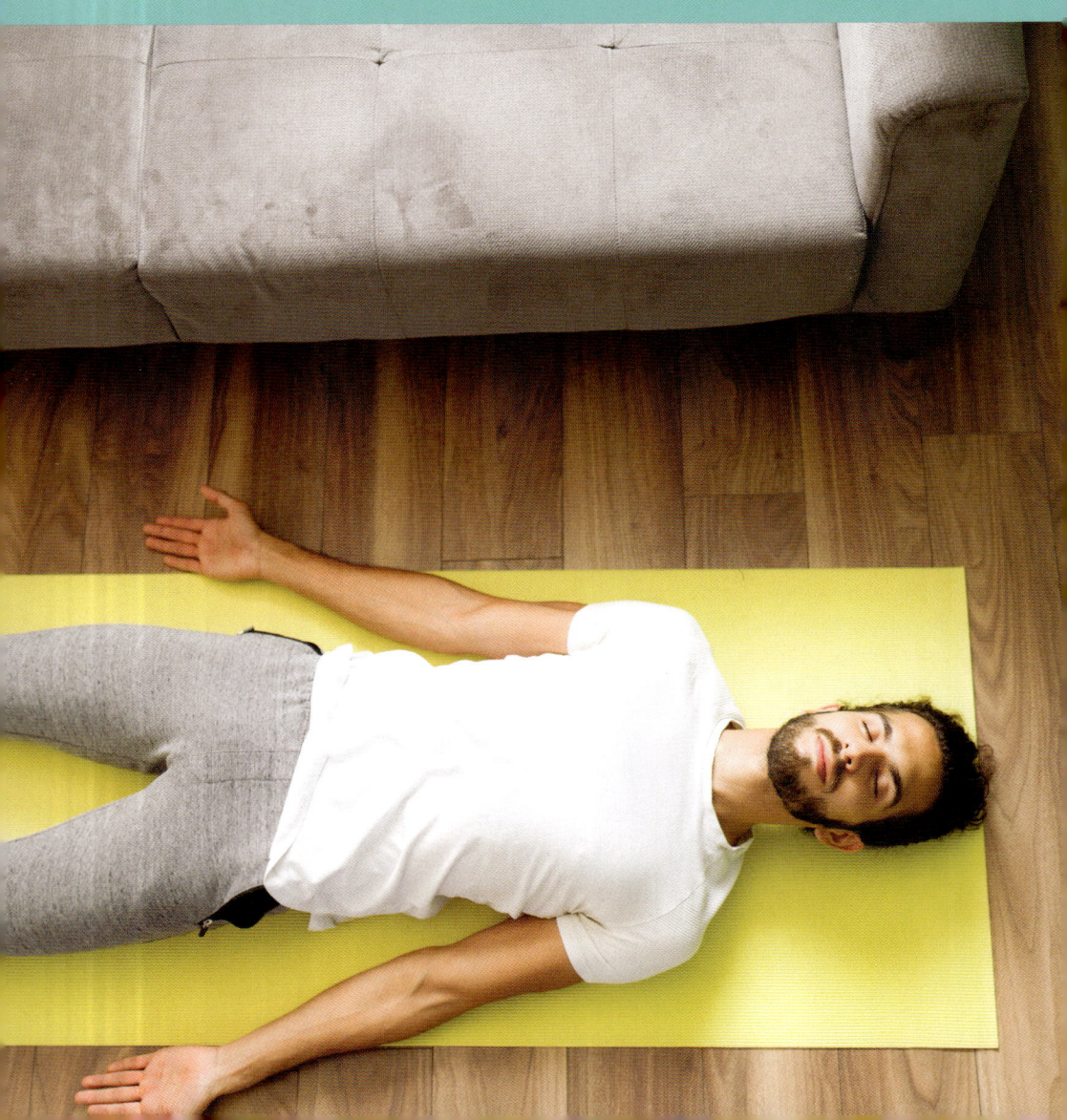

SLEEP FOR PEAK PERFORMANCE

Sleep is essential for sports performance, emotional regulation and recovery from fatigue. For footballers, adequate sleep is critical for both physical and mental health. Insufficient sleep, characterised by reduced duration and poor quality, can significantly increase the risk of illness and injury. Managing sleep and wake times to maintain a healthy circadian rhythm (the natural internal process that regulates the sleep-wake cycle) is vital, as disruptions to our biological clock can negatively affect sleep quality and overall athletic performance.

HOW YOGA ENHANCES SLEEP QUALITY

Yoga is increasingly recognised for its positive impact on sleep quality, particularly among athletes. Incorporating yoga into your routine can greatly improve both sleep and overall wellbeing. The poses, movements and breathwork outlined in this book offer several benefits.

The restorative poses, especially those in the relaxation routine, are highly effective in releasing muscular tension and preparing the body for restful sleep. Improved sleep quality aids in physical recovery by reducing inflammation and supporting tissue repair.

The focus on deep, slow breathing during yoga practice helps alleviate stress and anxiety. This is particularly beneficial during high-pressure periods such as heavy training loads and intense competition schedules. By calming the mind, you can enhance your sleep quality, which in turn improves your cognitive function and decision-making, allowing you to stay focused and tranquil despite external pressures.

INTEGRATING YOGA FOR OPTIMAL WELLBEING

Yoga balances your hormones by reducing cortisol levels, the stress hormone that can inhibit sleep, and enhancing melatonin production, which regulates sleep-wake cycles. Balanced hormones contribute to improved recovery, reduced stress and increased physical relaxation, leading to more restorative sleep.

This holistic approach supports athletic performance, injury prevention and overall health, underscoring the essential role of sleep in achieving peak performance and maintaining mental and physical health. Incorporating yoga routines into your daily practice can significantly enhance your sleep quality and overall wellbeing.

REFERENCES

Arbo, G. D. et al., 'Mitigating the antecedents of sports-related injury through yoga', *International Journal of Yoga*, 13(2) (2020), pp. 120–29.

Askling, C. M. et al., 'Acute first-time hamstring strains during high-speed running: A longitudinal study including clinical and magnetic resonance imaging findings', *The American Journal of Sports Medicine*, 35(2) (2007), pp. 197–206.

Askling, C. M. et al., 'Acute hamstring injuries in Swedish elite football: A prospective randomised controlled clinical trial comparing two rehabilitation protocols', *British Journal of Sports Medicine*, 47 (2013), pp. 953–59.

Askling, C. M. et al., 'Total proximal hamstring ruptures: Clinical and MRI aspects including guidelines for postoperative rehabilitation', *Knee Surgery, Sports Traumatology, Arthroscopy*, 21(3) (2013), pp. 515–33.

Candela, V., et al., 'Hip and groin pain in soccer players', *Joints*, 7(4) (2021), pp. 182–87.

Ekstrand, J. et al., 'Epidemiology of muscle injuries in professional football', *The American Journal of Sports Medicine*, 39(6) (2011), pp. 1226–32.

Gothe, N. P. et al., 'Yoga effects on brain health: A systematic review of the current literature', *Brain Plasticity*, 5(1) (2019), pp. 105–22.

Hausswirth, C. and Le Meur, Y., 'Physiological and nutritional aspects of post-exercise recovery: Specific recommendations for female athletes', *Sports Medicine*, 41(10) (2011), pp. 861–82.

Huang, K. and Ihm, J., 'Sleep and injury risk', *Current Sports Medicine Reports*, 20(6) (2021), pp. 286–90.

Kaminoff, L., *Yoga Anatomy* (Human Kinetics, 2007)

Kartal, A. and Ergin E., 'Investigation of the effects of 6-week Yoga exercises on balance, flexibility, and strength in soccer players', *International Journal of Human Movement and Sports Sciences*, 8(3) (2020), pp. 91–96.

Krishnamurthy, M. N., 'Yoga as part of sports medicine and rehabilitation', *International Journal of Yoga*, 16(2) (2023), pp. 61–63.

Milewski, M. D. et al., 'Chronic lack of sleep is associated with increased sports injuries in adolescent athletes', *Journal of Pediatric Orthopedics*, 34(2) (2014), pp. 129–33.

Polsgrove, M. J. et al., 'Impact of 10-weeks of yoga practice on flexibility and balance of college athletes', *International Journal of Yoga*, 9(1) (2016), pp. 27–34.

Sakai, Y., *Low Back Pain Pathogenesis and Treatment* (IntechOpen, 2012)

REFERENCES

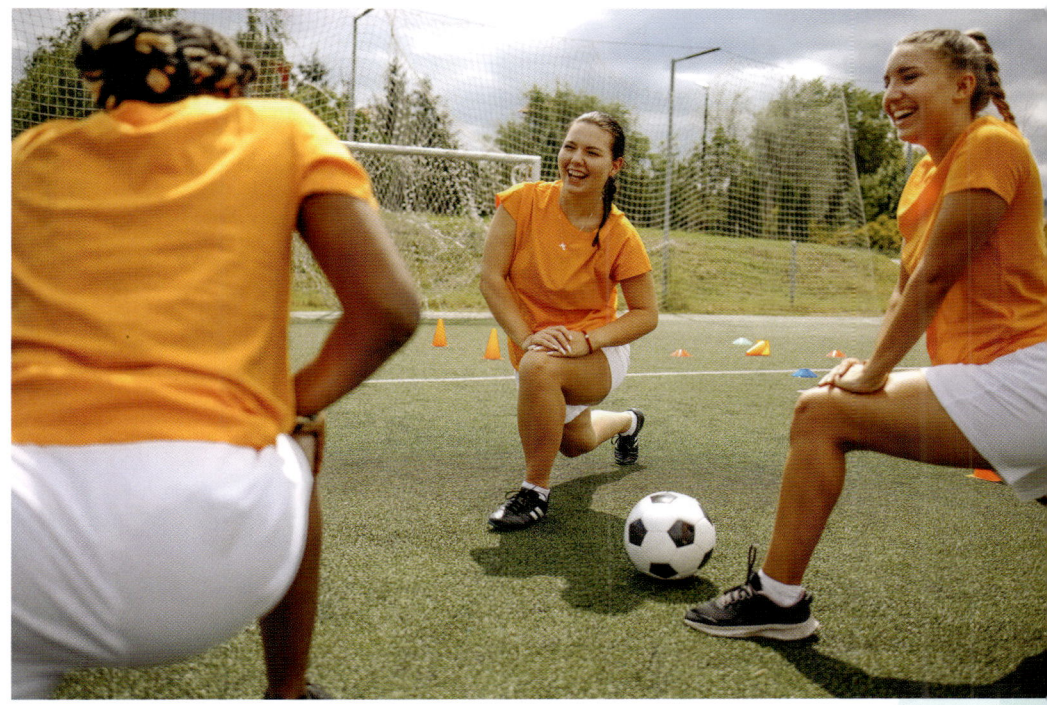

Schache, A. G. et al., 'Mechanics of the human hamstring muscles during sprinting', *Medicine and Science in Sports and Exercise*, 44(4) (2012), pp. 647–58.

Sherry, M. A. and Best, T. M., 'A comparison of 2 rehabilitation programs in the treatment of acute hamstring strains', *Journal of Orthopaedics and Sports Physical Therapy*, 34(4) (2004), pp. 116–25.

Sivananda Yoga Center, *The Sivananda Companion to Yoga* (Simon & Schuster, 2000)

Sivananda Yoga Center, *Yoga: Mind & Body* (DK Living, 1998)

Vieira de Castro, J., et al., 'Incidence of decreased hip range of motion in youth soccer players and response to a stretching program: A randomized clinical trial', *Journal of Sport Rehabilitation*, 22(2) (2013), pp. 100–7.

Volpi, P., *Football Traumatology: Current Concepts from Prevention to Treatment* (Springer, 2006)

ACKNOWLEDGEMENTS

Writing this book has been a lifelong dream. For as long as I can remember, I've had it attached to my vision boards, written down in journals and sticky notes, and it feels as though I've always been visualising and imagining it.

For years, the idea of putting my thoughts onto paper felt like a distant possibility – something I would do 'one day'. But life has a way of leading us to exactly what we desire, even when we don't expect it.

When the opportunity to write this book came my way, it arrived just as I was navigating a challenging chapter in my business. Life will open new doors when we find the courage to close old ones. In that space of uncertainty, this book became more than just a project. It reminded me why I started this journey with Football Yoga in the first place: to make a meaningful, global shift in football culture. This reminder gave me energy, purpose and a renewed sense of fulfillment, for which I am incredibly grateful.

First and foremost, my deepest gratitude goes to my daughter, Luna Rose. At just five years old, you have shown more patience than I could have ever asked for. The hours I spent writing meant time away from you, yet you embraced it with so much love and understanding. Your laughter, energy and hugs gave me strength and kept me going. I love you deeply, and I hope that as you grow, you will always know how much you inspire me.

To my parents, your tireless support has been my rock. Thank you for believing in me, even when I doubted myself. Not only did you encourage me throughout this journey, but you also stepped in to help with Luna Rose in so many ways, allowing me the time and space to bring this book to life. I could not have done this without you, and I am endlessly grateful for your constant love and generosity.

To Caroline, Holly and the entire publishing team at Bloomsbury, thank you for seeing something in me and reaching out with this opportunity. Your belief in my work and your guidance throughout this process have meant everything. From our first conversation to the final touches, you helped turn an idea into something tangible, and I am incredibly grateful to have had you by my side on this journey.

To my family, friends and everyone who checked in on me throughout this process, thank you. Whether it was a message of encouragement, a reminder to take a break, or simply being there to root for me, your support meant more than you know.

And finally, to you – the footballers, coaches, parents, match officials and everyone in the football community who has picked up this book – thank you. The world of football is constantly evolving, and I truly believe that integrating yoga into the game can transform not only performance, but also mindset, recovery, and overall physical and mental well-being. I hope this book brings value to your journey and helps you to discover new ways to move, breathe and play at your best.

This journey has been one of resilience, growth and gratitude. I am so thankful I kept the vision alive, and even more thankful that this book will play a small part in supporting those in the football world and beyond.

INDEX

alternate nostril breathing 149
asanas *see* poses
Askling L-Protocol 104

bananasana 153
bee breath 150
benefits 16–18
bird dog 136
blanket, yoga 21
boat 137
bolster, yoga 20
breathwork 14, 147
  alternate nostril breathing 149
  bee breath 150
  box breathing 39
  and cat and cow 28
  diaphragmatic breath 148
  4-7-8 breathing 83
bricks/blocks, yoga 21
bridge 124–5

cat and cow 28, 88
child's pose 80
  to cobra flow 130–1
clothing 19
cobra 50
  child's pose to 130–1
  downward-facing dog to cobra 51–2
  press-ups 129
core routine 133–45

dead bug movement 134
diagonal dynamic pigeon 63
diaphragmatic breath 148
dolphin 144
downward-facing dog 48–9
  to cobra flow 51–2
dynamic stretching 15, 16
  diagonal dynamic pigeon 63
  figure of eight 29, 69
  football yoga flow 57
  high lunge flow 55–6
  sun salutation 35

eccentric exercises 104
equipment 19–21
evening routine 75–83
the extender 104–5

figure of eight 29, 69
fish
  half lord of the 100–1
  supported 152
flexibility 15, 16
flows, defined 23
focus, mental 18
football star 54
football yoga flow 57
forward bend with twists 70–1
4-7-8 breathing 83
frog 94–5
  half 67–8

Giggs, Ryan 12
groin strains 61, 78, 87

half frog 67–8
half lord of the fish 100–1
half split (toes up and down) 64–5, 114–15
hamstring injuries 103
hamstring routine 103–17
hamstring strap stretch 116–17
health concerns 39, 45, 56
high lunge flow 55–6
hip routine 87–101

injury prevention 18, 87

joint mobility and stability 16–17

kidney function 30

lactic acid 59, 61, 81
legs up the wall 81–2
letter M movements 66
listen to your body 23
lizard 92–3

locust 127
low lunge cactus arms 123
lower back routine 119–31
lunge variations 38
lymphatic system 27, 30, 59

mat, yoga 20
mindfulness 17
mobility, joint 16–17
modified gate 61–2
morning routine 27–39
muscle massage 31

namaste 36–7, 42–3, 106–7
neck stretches 32
90/90 with movement 89

one-legged dog flow 142–3
oxygen exchange 83

parasympathetic nervous system 70, 83
   and breathwork 147, 148
pause for thought 23
performance 17–18
pigeon 79
   with twists 90–1
plank 44–5
   side 46–7
poses, defined 23
post-training/post-match routine 59–73
pre-training/pre-match routine 41–57
prevention, injury 7, 18, 155
proprioception 38, 136
pyramid 108–9

reclined butterfly 78
recovery 17, 59
   see also post-training/post-match routine
rehabilitation 8, 12, 103
   bird dog 136
   bridge 124
   dead bug movement 134
   the extender 104–5

relaxation 17, 18
relaxation routine 147–53
restorative postures 147
   bananasana 153
   supported fish 152
   twisting crouching tiger 151
reversed tabletop 128
rock 'n' rolls 33, 126, 135
routines, defined 23

savasana 72–3
single arm/leg plank 138–9
sleep 155
spinal dance 60, 120
stability, joint 16–17, 18
standing forward bend with twists 112–13
standing spinal twist 30–1
straps, yoga 21
stretching 15
sun salutation 34–5
supine twist 77
supported fish 152

thoracic book opening 76
thread the needle 121–2
tree 98–9
twisting crouching tiger 151

warrior 1 96–7
warrior 2 145
warrior 3 53
wide-legged forward bend with twists 110–11

yoga, origins 13–14
yoga plank 44–5
yoga side plank 46–7, 140–1